DOES THE BIBLE
TEACH NUTRITION?

Elizabeth Baker

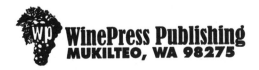

WinePress Publishing
MUKILTEO, WA 98275

Published by Winepress Publishing
PO Box 1406
Mukilteo, WA 98275

Cover by **DENHAM**DESIGN, Everett, WA

ISBN: 1-57921-035-X
Library of Congress Catalog Card Number: 97-60974

CONTENTS

INTRODUCTION

Some time ago I wrote an article at the suggestion of an editor friend of mine, which he entitled "Is Nutrition Taught in the Bible?" His idea proved to be a good one, for response to that article exceeded any previous response. It touched a keynote among his readers; it was a vital interest switch that lit up a sleeping giant, much neglected. It also touched something in me. I, too, was interested in what the Bible said about how to eat and what to eat, and began the rather long, sometimes tedious, fascinating study of the Bible. I must hit the high spots, I said to myself. I must emphasize them so people can see how important it is for us to recognize, understand and heed them, because *eating wrongly causes great harm to our bodies.*

Deep into my Bible research project I labored over fresh and engrossing ways to tell the familiar stories that deal with foods. Daniel's eating of pulse must be explained, then that of Moses and the children of Israel living on manna, and so on. I must bring into focus the little-known bits and pieces about nutrition scattered throughout the Bible, **such as the rarely quoted Proverbs that apply to eating.** There are many gems concerning food that are overlooked, and phrases about correct nourishment that are overshadowed by other truths, oft-quoted and memorized.

Once I was embarked on this new approach to the Bible as a textbook on nutrition, I "dug in." Much to my amazement, I found a wealth of material I had completely overlooked. Finding it scattered throughout the Old and New Testaments, I struggled to get it in some sort of order. The bits and pieces all through that marvelous book were at first like a great basketful of colorful mini-tiles displayed seemingly without organization. I toiled and prayed "without ceasing." Little by little, the first few tiles dropped into place, then others and still others. I began to see some order coming about. Always there is order in all God does and has us do. The outline of a plan started to appear. Pieces began to touch, to relate to each other, and spaces filled in. What finally, slowly emerged was a mosaic of God's teachings on how and what to eat. Right there in the Bible it is ready to remind us so we can obey His commands: the truths that can set us free from sickness and disease.

Chapter One

DO THE SCRIPTURES REALLY TEACH NUTRITION?

"Know ye not that ye are the temple of God, and that the Spirit of God dwelleth in you? If any man defileth the temple of God, him shall God destroy; for the temple of God is holy, which temple ye are" (I Corinthians 3:16–17).

From birth to death, God dealt with every aspect of life in His Scriptures. He provided the clearest teaching possible for the benefit of His beloved children. One teaching in particular is threaded all through the Bible in each and every book. Yet this all-important teaching is the most neglected, the most ignored of all Scriptural truths. It is the teaching on nutrition: what to eat, how much to eat and why.

In the very first chapter of the first book of the Bible God gave us His first commandment: *"Then God said, 'I give you every seed-bearing plant on the face of the whole* earth and every tree that has fruit with seed in it. They will be yours for food'" (Genesis 1:28–29, NIV).

The Garden of Eden had all manner of fruits and delicious edible plants. We know this for several reasons, one of them being that God would not have focused His first commandment on food without providing it in abundance. With that first commandment, He clearly described the food growing not only in the garden but over all the earth. It is a profound teaching on what we are to eat in words so simple, so clear, that any child can understand them. Yet it is singularly curious that almost all people who believe the Bible rarely think about these words as referring to nutrition. And if they do, they do not accept the instruction as applicable to themselves. They try to follow the Word of God, beginning with the Ten Commandments and continuing through the teachings of Jesus to the end of Revelation. However, the vast majority of us do not even see this first commandment. Or we ignore it, or consider it unimportant. We overlook it, or think it does not apply to us today.

This neglected commandment holds a prominent place in the *first chapter* of the *first book* of the Bible. How it can be so overlooked has to be among the greatest mysteries of all time.

Yet the Creator could not have made His commandment more understandable: herbs (leaves and vegetables) and their seeds, such as spinach, parsley, lettuces, squash, peppers, melons, tomatoes, cucumbers, legumes and grains; and fruits of trees bearing seeds, such as apples, oranges, papayas, plums and apricots. The seeds of these are edible and necessary in the small quantities the fruits provide for our total health. Yes, even papaya seeds are edible.

Man was created a vegetarian, with intestines three times as long as that of a carnivore of equal size, with a stomach ten times less acidic than a carnivore's, and with the biting, grinding, pulverizing teeth of a plant-eating animal. There was no word whatsoever about cooking God's wonderful food. Why would He have his people kill those fresh, living plants, destroying half their vitamins, minerals, enzymes and oxygen and leaving needless, useless waste for the body to dispose of? He made no provision for treating with heat what the entire animal kingdom, including man, ate during that period. Men, like the animals, ate their food raw.

From the time of Adam and Eve's disobedience and expulsion from the Garden to the time of Noah and the Flood, people ate as God had commanded. There is no record from that time of illness or disease, except Job's affliction which God allowed Satan to put upon him. On that diet people lived well over nine hundred years.

Another thing translators and scholars, Bible readers and followers have mainly overlooked or taken for granted is the most important of all nutrients. Well provided for mankind until recently, it has mainly been recognized only in the last century. It is one of the nutrients destroyed by cooking temperatures of 212 degrees and above. That nutrient is oxygen. We can live months without food, days without water, but only a few minutes without oxygen. Oxygen is the primary nutrient of all living things. *"And the Lord formed man of the dust of the ground, and breathed into his nostrils the breath of life; and man became a living soul"* (Genesis 2:7). The life-giving substance in the breath is oxygen.

According to research conducted by Dr. Carl Baugh, curator or the Creation Museum in Glenrose, Texas, there were no oceans covering the earth during the earliest time of Genesis. The people lived in very fertile valleys three miles below what is today sea level, on or near the bottom of what are known now as oceans.

Here is the account given by Moses in the Bible: *"And God said, Let there be a firmament [atmosphere] in the midst of [between] the waters, and let it divide the waters from the waters...And God made the firmament, and divided the waters which were under the firmament from the waters which were above the firmament: and it was so. And God called the firmament Heaven. And the evening and the morning were the second day. And God said, Let the waters under the heaven be gathered together unto one place, and let the dry land appear: and it was so. And God called the dry land Earth . . . "* (Genesis 1:6–10).

So perfect was the heavily oxygenated air in a climate neither too hot nor too cold that man, plants and animals grew to enormous sizes and lived a long time. Man lived to be nearly a thousand years old. Heavier air pressure than we have today and abundant oxygen were major reasons for his long lifespan. Also, in an atmosphere of bounteous oxygen, bacteria, viruses, amoebae, molds, decay and fermentation could not exist. Add the factors of the heavier air pressure and the greater amount of oxygen to the pristine water and the natural, live foods he ate, and it becomes understandable why man's lifespan was over twelve times as long as it is today. He had twelve times as many good things going for him. He was without illness. When mankind and all other forms of life took in more oxygen, they were *disease free,* lived longer and had greater strength, health and endurance. Oxygen was and is, truly, nutrient number one.

These were some of the reasons man grew larger and was highly intelligent, being able to use all of his magnificent brain as described in Genesis by Moses. Today we use only a part of our brains, mainly because we take in less oxygen. But man, after being expelled from Eden, increasingly used his great intelligence for evil. All but Noah and his family turned away from God to go their wicked ways. God was grieved and regretted that He had made man. But because there was one righteous person, Noah, He told him to build the ark for himself and family and all the animals. The huge boat was finished by the time God allowed the Flood to come to cleanse the earth and to destroy all except what went into the ark. Only Noah, his wife, his three sons and their wives, seven pairs of each of the clean animals and creatures, and a single pair of each of the unclean ones went into the ark and survived the great deluge. Since food was scarce, God probably permitted the eating of the flesh of the clean animals. However, it was not cooked but was eaten raw as the animals ate their food. Noah, his family and all the animals and creatures came out of the ark to a bare world, devoid of vegetation. There might have been some roots for food, but mostly they had to eat flesh until vegetation appeared on the earth, no doubt a matter of months or years.

Why did man' lifespan shorten steadily after the Flood to 120 years, as recorded in Genesis 6:3? Although there were several reasons, one in particular stands out. Scientists have recently brought that reason to light through new discoveries, analytical thinking, observations and calculations. Prior to the Flood the great canopy of water vapor above the atmosphere in outer space completely covered the earth like a mighty glass globe. This canopy was made up of two layers of water with a thin, transparent, crystalline layer of metal in between. This crystalline layer shielded the earth from the ultraviolet rays of the sun. Since ultraviolet rays are harmful, this protection alone could have helped to account for the long life of man before the Flood.

The vapor ring was maintained in its place miles high above the atmosphere by centrifugal energy. Warm rays of the sun penetrated the watery covering to give the sky a beautiful azure blue, creating a perfect light. In this ideal climate where neither extreme heat nor extreme cold ever occurred, drastic upheavals of nature, such as hurricanes, earthquakes and storms, never disturbed the quiet that enveloped the earth. It was in this ideal greenhouse-like atmosphere that man lived so long. The soil yielded luscious plants in great abundance and animals lived so long and well on the ideal forage that they reached enormous sizes, even up to ninety feet in length.

Before the Flood man lived three miles below the level of the present day seas formed by the deluge. At that depth, air pressure was approximately twenty-eight pounds per square inch. After the Flood all life lived three miles higher, and air pressure was approximately 14.73 pounds per square inch. (Atmospheric pressure lowers with each mile higher above sea level and increases somewhat proportionately with each mile lower down.) The higher pressure of twenty-eight pounds per square inch caused the atmosphere to be between 40 percent and 50 percent oxygen. The lower pressure of 14.73 pounds per square inch caused the atmosphere to be between 30 percent and 35 percent oxygen.

From the time God created the heavens and the earth until the Flood, the earth was watered by a mist rising from the earth and moisture rising from below the surface of the ground. There was no rain. Storms never occurred to disturb the quiet that enveloped the earth. In this perfect

12

atmosphere, no wonder man lived more than nine hundred years!

The mighty Flood, from the fall of the great covering of water, poured down millions of tons of water in the short span of forty days and forty nights. Over seventy-one percent of the earth's surface was left covered with water after the downpour ceased, and the receding waters leveled to form our present day seas. Only the original high peaks and mountain plateaus were left, thrusting above the water and forming the earth's six continents of today.

Chapter Two

CAN FOODS DETERMINE THE LENGTH OF OUR LIFESPAN?

During the time of the earth's reconstruction and the Flood family's adjustment to it, Noah planted a vineyard. In due time he harvested his first yield. As was the custom, he juiced the fruit and set his jars of nectar in the storage shelter, then took his ease and drank of the fruits of his crop. What was unknown at the time was the fact that, due to the lower oxygen content of the air, a new process had been born—the process now known as fermentation. His juice had fermented and created alcohol. Not knowing anything of this development, he drank his fill of the sparkling, different-tasting nectar and became drunk. It was a totally new experience for him. Poor old Noah was completely innocent of any wrongdoing. What was a sin was the way his son Ham burst in on his naked father, then ran to tell (some say "blab") his brothers. Nakedness was a strictly private matter and to be respected. Shem and Japheth, Noah's other sons, showed their respect by backing into their father's room with a garment laid across their shoulders and covering his nakedness. (See Genesis 9:23.)

Now, more about the shortening lifespan of man. We can begin to understand why it could actually drop from nearly one thousand years to 120 years in only ten generations when we review the awesome things that happened all at once: (1) bacteria, virus, disease, mold, fermentation and decay came into being; (2) the diet was changed from God-intended vegetarianism to emergency fare, mainly the eating of flesh; (3) oxygen in the air was greatly reduced. (Not only was there less oxygen to breathe, but there was less oxygen in the foods and water man ate and drank.) Questions naturally surface. How does a drop in oxygen due to lowered air pressure so drastically cut the lifespan? The *amount* of oxygen, scientists believe, holds much of the answer.

Remember that God designed man with powerful lungs to live mightily in an atmospheric pressure of around twenty-eight pounds per square inch and an oxygen content of between 40 percent and 50 percent. Those lungs could withstand and take in oxygen-saturated air to fill the great chest with each breath. By breathing this large amount of cleansing oxygen, all body wastes were so completely removed that the blood was pure. When the blood is pure, the health is excellent.

Remember also what happened in an atmosphere of 40 percent to 50 percent oxygen: there were no viruses, bacteria, amoebae, molds, fermentation or decay, and therefore no disease, no infections. Actually, God made the human being to live forever. If man had continued in God's perfect will, he would have done so. But he disobeyed, be-

16

coming imperfect with evil in his nature, and was turned out of the garden into a world that became imperfect because of Adam and Eve's sin. Even so, he still lived nine hundred plus years. But after having to live at an elevation three miles higher, with much less air pressure and oxygen, his large lungs, capable of handling the original abundant amount of life-giving, health-maintaining oxygen, he was able to get only about two-thirds of the original amount of oxygen. The air pressure was not sufficient to force the breath of deep breathing to fill the lungs. With only 30 percent oxygen in the air, the blood could not be optimally purified of toxins from body wastes. Keep in mind that life is in the blood. The purer the blood, the better the health. The more impure the blood, the poorer the health and the sicker the body.

To summarize the oxygen story through history:

- 40% to 50% oxygen in the air before the Flood
- 30% to 35% oxygen in the air after the Flood
- 25% to 29% oxygen in the air after 1900
- 23% oxygen in the air in America up to the 1950s
- 18% or 19% oxygen in the air in America in the 1990s
- 17% down to 10% oxygen in towns and cities in America today

For the majority of our citizenry, there remains approximately half the oxygen we had before the turn of the century. With a deficiency of oxygen alone, the national health averages would be down. Add to that, polluted water and air; chemically treated plants, crops and produce of all kinds; disease and parasite-infested, chemically treated, commercially raised poultry and meat; artificial, processed, nutrient-robbed products; irradiated and microwave-zapped foods; and mineral-depleted, chemically fertilized, crop-dusted and sprayed soils. It all gives a grim picture of today's world.

The food God commanded us to eat was fresh, living, wholesome and natural, full of oxygen which enabled that food to be optimally utilized by the body. It also kept the body clean and free of toxins. That food was raw, not destroyed by heat (cooking) which, on an average, destroys half the food value. Both before and after the Flood and until the time of Moses, people did not cook food. Being full of oxygen, it could give near-total health. And their diets were vegetarian, complete in proteins and fats (seeds and nuts), in carbohydrates (primarily in seeds, nuts, grains, and fruits), and in minerals, abundant in fruits.

After the Flood and because of the destruction of plants from the Flooding, God provided generously for Noah and his family by having ordered into the ark seven pairs of clean, edible animals. Of the unclean ones, He had ordered only one pair of each to enter. He was very careful to instruct Noah (and succeeding generations) what flesh not to eat and why. Forbidden flesh included crustaceans—fish without scales (scavenger shellfish) living at the bottom of large bodies of water, where they help keep the waters clean and survive on dead food. Scavenger birds who eat dead, decaying flesh, and certain animals, like pigs, camels and hares, were prohibited as well because their flesh harbors parasites. The approved flesh, such as cattle, sheep and deer, was primarily eaten raw, as flesh-eating animals eat it.

Beginning with the time of Moses centuries later, when God brought His laws and the burnt sacrifices and offerings of animals into being, cooked flesh was introduced to all the people. The odor was so pleasant that they soon got the taste and craving for it. (Cooked flesh is powerfully addictive.) This helped to bring the lifespan down from 120 years to seventy to eighty years. *"The days of our years are threescore years and ten; and if by reason of strength they be fourscore years, yet is their strength labor and sorrow..."* (Psalm 90:10).

Cooking among the Hebrews really began when Joseph brought his people into Egypt at the invitation of Pharaoh. Then after the exodus from Egypt some of them ground and cooked the manna that God provided and had intended for His people to eat fresh every day, and uncooked.

Couple the scarcity of oxygen in the atmosphere with its scarcity in cooked food and the scarcity in water we get by drinking coffee, tea and carbonated drinks. None of these drinks have oxygen. Most people drink little good, fresh water. One begins to realize that every person, indeed every creature on the face of the earth, is half-starved for this life-sustaining gas called oxygen. It is a great wonder that man lives as long and as functionally as he does. It is a greater wonder that man has any health at all when one considers the leached, over-farmed soils, the herbicides, the pesticides, the genetically and hormonally altered vegetables, fruits, seeds and grains of today.

Oxygen plays an all-important part in sickness and ill health. Cancer cells, for instance, are anaerobic, meaning this: they proliferate only where cells get no oxygen. It is much the same with all degenerative diseases that cannot thrive where cells receive a normal amount of oxygen, because these diseases are anaerobic. If sufficient oxygen is supplied to all the cells, they will not become diseased. If at the same time the cells are nourished with pure water and natural, unaltered foods, those cells are kept clean and free of waste and body filth, then the body can function with radiant health and vigor.

Even in the time before Noah, God provided completely for man's physical well-being, then gave him full instructions for eating right to keep his body healthy and clean. The fresh, living foods and the pure water were as well oxygenated as the air itself. In every way man got far more oxygen into his body and bloodstream than he does today. Since oxygen is the most cleansing agent on the earth, it must be given top priority in the care and feeding of our body. *"If any man defile the temple of God, him shall God destroy; for the temple of God is holy, which temple ye are"* (I Corinthians 3:17).

Since junk foods—overcooked, processed, chemical-laden and artificial—have no oxygen, they are harmful to God's temple, the temple of our soul-spirit. To eat them day by day is bit by bit to destroy that temple, the only body we have. It displeases Him because it is wrong. It ignores His teaching. It prematurely allows the body to age and deteriorate. Such eating is in disobedience to God. It is a sin.

Is it any wonder that the United States is the sickest developed nation in the world? The wonder is that we function as healthily as we do, especially when we face the reality of universal oxygen deficiency. Mankind, plants and animals—all living things—are oxygen-starved. Being oxygen starved, we are riddled by disease. The plagues prophesied for the end times are upon us, make no mistake: AIDS, the new deadly, mutated tuberculosis virus, the *E. coli* virus (and lately new and even deadlier *E. coli*-type viruses in

South and Central America, Africa and Japan), death-causing parasites, and so on. I believe parasites are among the pestilences spoken of in the Scriptures. There are many, well over a hundred kinds already identified, new parasites from all over the world and old ones we've known about for years. It is estimated by parasitologists that there are around a thousand parasites. They range in size from the large tape worm to the microscopic fluke. Recently, it has been discovered that when parasites have been in a body for some time, viruses find their way to them, attach themselves, and live in or on those parasites and they infect the infecting parasites (a parasite in or on a parasite). Viruses can and do live on bacteria. In professional vernacular it is called "piggybacking."

God promises to protect us from the plagues (diseases, pestilences) of the end times if we keep His commandments. Taking the responsibility for our own health, making the effort to find out how and what to eat, and treating the temple of our soul-spirit the way God wishes are all a part of God's commandments. When we keep *all commandments*, we can claim that promise. He will protect us from end-time plagues and pestilences.

Chapter Three

How Far Have We Strayed from God in Our Eating?

The fascinating story line of Genesis carries us through the "lesser" verses which are soon dismissed by many as applying only to the times of Eden and the Flood. God's several instructions about food are in keeping with His powerful yet loving character, and are given with simplicity, force and economy of words. It's incredible that those words are taken for granted by many of us. God was the great provider of everything. Food was a natural part of it all, but foods, say people today, have changed long since then. Indeed they have, but God and His word have not changed.

A commonly held opinion is that God now provides different foods for man because times are different, and of course they are. An opinion not infrequently expressed is that God gave man the intelligence to do new things, to develop products for the betterment of mankind. This is true. But man has too often used this intelligence, this gift of invention and creativity for wrong purposes, for unfair gain, for greed, and even for criminal evil as was done in the times of Noah. Alterations of foods, destruction of nutrients, and use of false and harmful substances at the expense of the consumer and for the financial benefit of the manufacturer/processor hold the answers to many of our diseases. A review of Biblical history (see Genesis 1:29) tells us from where we have gone astray and so have destroyed our health. Opinions aside, the answer boils down to one stark basic truth: We have gotten away from the *natural* in our lives. We have unbelievably increased in knowledge while pulling away from our foundation, our roots. As in the days of Noah, we are using much of it unwisely, for evil purposes, for personal gain at the expense of the whole of mankind. We are not heeding the Almighty's counsel, nor are we teaching it anywhere except in health centers, a few universities, an occasional clinic, or random classes and scattered lectures by nutrition-minded people. It is only beginning to be mentioned in Bible teaching.

To see what other factors may have contributed to the low state of our national health, let's look at a story in the life of many of us alive today. In the 1950s, as I wrote earlier, oxygen in the air was 23 percent. By the 1990s it was down to 18 and 19 percent in the open country, and 17 percent down to 10 percent in populated areas. That means we have available to us only about one half the amount of oxygen we need in order to sustain a truly healthy body and mind.

Shouldn't we begin to see why we have so much illness and disease in our world today? The lowering of the oxygen, combined with the ever present threat and danger—the toxicity in the air we breathe—can make for a harrowing experience every time we inhale!

At least we can understand how man's lifespan steadily decreased to 120 years over a period of ten generations in the years following the Flood. Not only less oxygen but a largely overlooked factor helped bring this shortened life about: the eating of much flesh. As in the animal kingdom where flesh eaters live shorter lives, so among men the eating of too much flesh shortens the lifespan.

There will always be opinions and differences of opinion. But when people can give good reasons and show positive results from certain ways of thinking and doing things, they have valid criteria for their case.

Our opinion is based on the original plan for Adam and Eve. They were to enjoy perfect health in the Garden of Eden where lush vegetation abounded, providing in easy access all the food they needed, ready to eat. There was no sickness or death. *"And God said, Let the earth bring forth grass, the herb yielding seed, and the fruit after his kind, whose seed is in itself, upon the earth . . . "* (Genesis 1:11).

Health without blemish and perfect contentment were the design for them. They had only to eat the vegetation God provided.

We read on: *". . . Everything that has the breath of life in it—I give every green plant for food . . . "* (Genesis 1:30, NIV). That includes us all. We have the breath of life in us.

"And the Lord God made all kinds of trees grow out of the ground—trees that were pleasing to the eye and good for food . . . " (Genesis 2:9). Everything originally created was beautiful.

When temptation came, curiosity and desire to taste (appetite) took over and Eve and her husband Adam gave in. How interesting to observe that both God's first commandment and man's first sin had to do with food. Because of this sin of disobedience, man is now vulnerable to both sickness and death.

The further we get from the *natural* (God), the more we get into trouble and suffer sickness. The Bible's words are clear on this point. The statement is simple and direct. *". . . If thou wilt diligently hearken to the voice of the Lord thy God, and wilt do that which is right in his sight, and wilt give ear to his commandments, and keep all his statutes, I will put none of these diseases upon thee, which I have brought upon the Egyptians: for I am the Lord that healeth thee"* (Exodus 15:26).

How abundantly clear God's words are on obeying His laws regarding diet and health! By observing them we may lessen and even avoid disease and so extend our lives. Certainly epidemic plagues are not God's will. *"Beloved, I wish above all things that thou mayest prosper and be in health, even as thy soul prospereth"* (III John 2).

For centuries, man from time to time has occupied himself most intently with the secret of physical life. Yet for centuries that secret has been available to the world in the simplest of terms. The prophets knew and wrote about it, and Moses gave us that knowledge in his account in Genesis of the first life upon the earth. Since that time the beginning of life remains the same for every person when he is born out of the womb of his mother: *". . . And [God] breathed into his nostrils the breath of life; and man became a living soul"* (Genesis 2:7).

The breath of life is oxygen, which we get from the air we breathe, the water we drink and the living foods we eat. Oxygen-rich food, well-oxygenated air and pure, fresh water nourish us and cleanse us of all toxins, including disease. The disease may have started from the waste of cooked, dead, oxygen-less, processed foods, from chemicals in what we eat and drink, or from pollution in the air we breathe and from medical drugs. The life-giving oxygen we take in and breathe enters through the lungs into the bloodstream to cleanse it, then it circulates to the cells to purify and nourish them. The nature of oxygen is to give life to the blood. As the prophets wrote, life is in the blood. That life is, first of all, oxygen, the *breath* of life.

Today the awesome power of the marvelous gas—oxygen—is the beginning, the fountainhead, the spring of all life. Oxygen saves countless critical care and emergency trauma patients. Oxygen can eliminate the symptoms of hang-over from alcohol abuse and is given in cases of coronary failure. One author in the fifties wrote: "Without it there could be no combustion, no fire. Every man, animal and plant would die and the earth become desolate and void!"

This is why every adult must learn about oxygen and take responsibility for getting more than just enough for survival. We must, every one, do everything possible to effect a change of lifestyle that can provide an optimal amount of oxygen to assure good health and well-being. Oxygen is the master key. To get enough today one must eat living foods rich in oxygen, drink pure water and exercise the body to increase the amount of oxygen taken in through the lungs.

This all can start with turning to our Lord and trusting Him for decisions and determination, then perseverance to put it into practice and patience to carry on while waiting for results. A failure to do so inevitably leads to disease, an accident-prone body and premature death. God doesn't desire that.

He wants us to remember that with plenty of oxygen getting to all the cells, cancer cells do not proliferate. Many professionals in the health field believe oxygen is a major answer to cancer.

Chapter Four

Why did Lifespans Greatly Shorten after the Flood?

From the beginning of biblical time to the Great Flood, God's people ate the food He provided for them. With no disease, affliction or infestation mankind lived for many generations. Can you imagine what it was like not being sick and living nearly a decade of centuries?

Those years, contrary to what some people say, were the same length then as they are today. The earth's course is set by the sun, determining the length of the days and the nights. The solar system since the beginning of Bible times is the same. The length of the year has not changed. It is still a little longer than 365 days, regardless of how a calendar may divide it into days, weeks and months. It has been the same in all ages and all countries. So man actually lived nearly a thousand years.

Why did such drastic changes in his number of days on Earth come about? There were reasons. Let's go back to the Bible to point out more of them.

We've already noted the changes in air pressure on the surface of the Earth from the time of Adam before the Flood and the time of Noah after the Flood. When mankind dwelt three miles lower down when there were no seas, he lived in such an amplitude of oxygen—the basic, necessary nutrient—that he enjoyed supreme health. He knew no physical, emotional or mental dysfunction. A totally adequate diet of fresh, natural foods and high oxygen in the air prevented it. Friendly, oxygen-thriving (aerobic) bacteria flourished to take care of body and plant waste. In the powerfully active oxygen-rich air, such natural refuse as feces and urine quickly disappeared.

With less than half as much oxygen in the world today, man uses roughly only half his lung capacity for regular breathing. Not only are his cells so starved that his body cannot last, for the most part, a hundred healthy years, the atmosphere is so low in oxygen that viruses, molds, bacteria, fermentation, rot and decay proliferate, threatening all life.

In other words, today we live in a disease-infested world.

A second reason for the lifespan being greatly shortened was change in diet. It came about after Moses was given the laws governing sacrifices and burnt offerings. Many people consider this reason controversial, but it need not be. There is proof to substantiate it.

Man started cooking most of the food God provided and originally meant to be eaten raw. *Living plants* are full of all the nutrients necessary for maintaining the body in the way He intended. Perhaps most importantly, living plants are full of oxygen, which assures the full utilization of vitamins, minerals, carbohydrates, proteins and fats necessary for optimal health, energy, strength, endurance and prevention of sickness and disease. When man applies fire—heat—which kills living food, he destroys nearly half the nutritional value in it. When he eats it, the nutritional needs of his body are only about half met. As a result, he suffers deficiencies. Taking all these factors into consideration, how can man's lifespan not be expected to diminish 40 percent, down from 120 years to seventy years?

Chapter Five

THE GREAT SHIFT
IN OUR FOOD CHOICE

What change in the nutritional realm followed the times of Moses? Besides more and more eating of meat, there was fire-baked bread of ground grains that largely replaced the bread made of sprouted grains (the pulse of Daniel's diet) and "baked" in the sun.

Flesh meat, slow to digest in the human system, putrefies before it is eliminated, causing toxins in the intestines to collect and be absorbed into the bloodstream. Cooked starch is another difficult-to-digest food. The starch (gluten) in wheat breads is the most difficult to digest of all cooked starches. There is gluten in rye, barley and oats, although much less than in wheat, triticale and spelt. By contrast, sprouted grains (pulse) are one of the easiest of foods to digest. In the germinating/budding/sprouting process, the starches are converted to fruit sugars and the proteins are converted to amino acids, also easy to digest. Actually, both of these sprout nutrients are predigested. Each

33

one makes almost no demands on the stomach, going directly into the upper intestines (duodenum) for the beginning process of absorption. Moreover, uncooked, raw, sprouted grains are rich in nutrients. They are fresh, full of oxygen and enzymes, as well as vitamins. They are truly life giving.

The word *pulse* means "flow of life." A nurse "takes our pulse" by feeling the blood being pumped through the arteries by the heart. This is the flow of life through the body by way of the blood stream. Sprouted seeds and grains flow with life after the dry, dormant seeds are activated by water. They are fresh, living, wholesome, natural and full of oxygen, enabling them to be optimally utilized by the body. They also keep the body clean and free of toxins. They are living, not killed by heat.

Both before and immediately after the Flood people did not cook. Food was totally health-giving. Until the Flood it was vegetarian, complete in proteins, fats, carbohydrates, enzymes, oxygen, vitamins and minerals. People ate mainly vegetarian fare from the time of Noah and the Flood until the time of Moses, centuries later, when God brought His laws—burnt sacrifices of animals—into being. The priests were given the savory-smelling meat to eat after the offering of it to the Lord. The odor of cooked flesh was pleasant, and people soon acquired a craving for it. Those who could afford flesh meat tended to overeat it.

Solomon eventually realized the problem. He explained it by calling meat deceitful because mankind was tempted to eat too much of it. *"Be not desirous of his [rulers' and officials'] dainties: for they are deceitful meat"* (Proverbs 23:3). *"Be not among winebibbers; among riotous eaters of flesh"* (Proverbs 23:20). *"The days of our years are three-*

score years and ten; and if by reason of strength they be fourscore years, yet is their strength labour and sorrow; for it is soon cut off, and we fly away" (Psalm 90:10). David, the Psalm writer, is saying in essence, "If one happens to have the strength to live to be eighty, that last decade of years is labored and sorrowful because of a failing body, ill health, old age fragility or perhaps senility."

The Israelites liked the smell of cooked flesh food. To them it was appetizing, much more so than the smell of raw meat. Scientists today realize how very persuasive is the sense of smell. It was so powerful the Israelites soon ate all flesh cooked. In fact, they began to cook almost everything they ate. Some were even cooking the manna God provided and originally intended to be eaten raw. The living plant food was full of all the nutrients necessary for the body in the way He intended and according to His commandment. Time and the experiences of various peoples and cultures have proven raw foods are health giving. Cooked foods are mainly only life sustaining.

By contrast, junk foods have no oxygen and the rest of the original nutrients are mostly destroyed. Those foods are more harmful than beneficial. To eat them displeases God because it is wrong and against His teaching. It is disobedience, a turning away from Scriptural truth and teaching. According to many leading physicians, junk foods, overeating and lack of oxygen, for whatever reasons, are the leading causes of sickness.

Today, more than ever, we must avoid eating dead foods. The flesh from a dead, butchered, dressed animal is *dead food.* There is no life force left in it, just as there is no life force left in us when our bodies die. The life force in fresh, raw plant food gives life, wellness and resistance to disease. Such foods are easily digested and assimilated because they contain all digestive aids, a main one being enzymes. With sufficient enzymes, the pancreas is not forced to overwork by having to manufacture enzymes to replace those lost in cooking and processing. If the foods are raw, they are complete. Whole. By eating them we, like the animals, can stay free of disease.

An interesting fact about digestive enzymes was discovered in the Philippines, where white rice makes up the bulk of the diet for countless low-income people. Researchers found that most adults in those areas over age forty have pancreases more than twice the normal size. Cooked white rice, containing no enzymes, requires the pancreas to overwork to produce enough enzymes to digest it, causing the pancreas to enlarge.

God does not condemn cooked food, nor are we under the covenant of the Old Testament which holds to the diet rules of not eating "unclean" flesh. One eats such things at his own risk. It has always been risky to eat shellfish, and much more so today because of pollution in the water, both fresh and sea. The Center for Disease Control in Atlanta reports that the incidence of hepatitis has increased ten times in the last decade. They attribute much of that increase to contaminated shellfish. It is well known and generally recognized that certain ethnic groups that follow a mainly vegetarian diet, much of it raw, maintain healthier lives and live longer.

If we look for proof of the efficacy of raw, living food in the diet, we have only to turn our attention to the animal kingdom. Animals do not process the foods they eat. They do not heat their food. Birds and some animals, such as squirrels that eat grains and seeds, allow the grains and seeds to soften by holding them in their craws or cheeks for several hours before they masticate and/or swallow them. This allows the grain to germinate, increasing the value of the food several times over in the process and making it easier to digest. Animals in their natural state usually live out their lives to the fullest extent if they are at the top of their food chain, which of course, is not cooked. Every cattleman knows that a young calf will live only about six weeks if fed pasteurized milk. In the heating to pasteurization temperature (180 degrees), too many micro-nutrients are destroyed to allow the milk to be life giving. On homogenized-pasteurized milk, a calf's life will be even shorter.

A few years ago Dr. Pottinger of Monrovia, California, demonstrated the effect of cooked and/or raw foods on cats. He divided some three dozen house cats into three groups. He fed one group all cooked foods. To another group he fed half cooked food, half raw. To the last group he fed only raw foods.

Much of the diet of all three groups was based on meat. The succeeding generations of cats in the first group became progressively weaker; they were quarrelsome, whiny, watery-eyed, narrow-faced; their fur was thin, uneven and dull. They could not reproduce after a few generations.

The cats in the second group fared better. They were moderately sociable cats, had acceptable coats of fur, had no trouble with reproduction or giving birth to normal, average cats.

The third group of cats was a sociable lot but fierce when challenged; they were quick footed; their faces were broader than their counterparts in the other groups; their jaws were better developed than either of the other groups; the size of their offspring was larger, more active and developed faster; their fur was thick, even and shiny. (Note:

A film of Dr. Pottenger's cats can be obtained from The Pottenger Foundation, Monrovia, California.)

Many athletes have found they have increased energy when they consume more fruits and vegetables in the raw state. One of the reasons for this is that cooked foods take longer to digest, thus requiring considerably more of one's total energy. For example, meat will stay in the intestines from forty to one hundred hours. All that time the body has to work hard to produce extra digestive juices and enzymes to break down the nutrients in the flesh meat for being assimilated. That work—digestion—requires a considerable expenditure of energy on the part of the body.

A conventional, mostly cooked meal of carbohydrates (starches such as bread, potatoes and vegetables) with a meat serving will take from 30 percent to 65 percent of the eater's total energy to digest. Not only does meat remain in the gut for many hours, but cooked starches are difficult and slow to digest, partly because they tend to impact in the bowel. During this time, the meat ingested invariably putrefies. In other words, it rots, the main cause of the bad odor of the feces.

On the other hand, a meal of raw fruits or vegetables along with nuts or seeds will take from 10 percent to 15 percent of the eater's total energy to process and requires sixteen to twenty-four hours for the body to eliminate. There are of course exceptions to these statements about raw vs. cooked foods, but they are few. The stories of those who adopt an all-natural, mostly raw foods-type of diet are the same: abundant energy, better-quality sleep, need for fewer hours of sleep in many cases, normal weight, a well-functioning body, a more alert mind and an uplifted, positive attitude.

Once people manage to make a change from conventional cooked and processed foods and commit themselves to staying with that commitment, they are greatly impressed with how much better they feel. They not only have more energy, but they experience a more joyous life.

Chapter Six

ARE WE TRULY
WHAT WE EAT?

L et's examine the statement about the United States being the most unhealthy of the developed nations in the world. To find out why, it is necessary to examine the foods we eat to see if they really are, as believed, the primary cause of our ignominious distinction in regard to health.

At the turn of the century, three major food products came on the market in sufficient quantity to supply the entire populace at prices families could afford to pay. They were white flour, white sugar and white vegetable shortening and oil. All had a long shelf life. Their taste, their stability and their versatility in cooking seemed perfect. But after ten years had passed, health problems began appearing across the nation—heart disease, varicose veins, arthritis, weight gain and diabetes, to mention some of the most life-threatening ones. With this upsurge of sickness, physicians began poring over research. Insulin was discovered in

1921 and diabetes diagnosed. Hypoglycemia, often a forerunner of diabetes, was diagnosed in 1922 but totally ignored for over forty years. Physicians found no dramatic "cure," as insulin was for diabetes.

What was it about these three highly processed foods that started the downward spiral in the health of United States of America? Medical science eventually realized what had happened. The new technology/processing stripped the foods of most of the vitamins, minerals and fiber (bulk). In the case of white flour, the bran containing vitamins and minerals and the germ of the wheat grain, containing essential oil and vitamin E, are taken out, leaving only *15 percent* of the original nutrition contained in whole grain flour. If you went to the bank to take out the one hundred dollars you had put in your savings account and they gave you only fifteen dollars, you would vehemently object and accuse them of robbery. When food is robbed, we say little or nothing.

In the processing of vegetable oils and margarine, vitamin E is destroyed, along with traces of other essential nutrients. Most of what is left after the hydrogenation process is very harmful to the body. Hydrogenation does to the oils just the opposite of what nature intended. Instead of helping to keep the veins and arteries free of hard fat and cholesterol deposits, these chemically treated oils and margarines "gum up" the blood vessels with sticky plaque, to which phospholipids (fats) and the bad (LDL) cholesterol stick. In other words, in the altered state, hydrogenated oils are foreign to and totally bad for the body. Biochemists have found they are one of the main causes of heart and blood vessel problems. Many doctors recognize this fact. These processed fats can sit on a shelf out of refrigeration for a hundred years and never go stale or rancid. There is almost no nutrition in them. No insect or animal will eat them. Man is the only creature on the earth that will.

As for refined white sugar, the processing that produces it removes everything but those naked crystals of pure calories. All the vitamins—B, C, A, D, E, etc.—and the macro and trace minerals are lost in processing . Many nutritionists call white sugar public enemy number one. People of all ages, from infancy to senility, eat it. Nothing is quite so addictive. It is the most overeaten of all food items, yet it is not really a food because it does not nourish. Immunologists have discovered that a sizable portion of sugar, like a candy bar or a sweet dessert, will literally shut down the immune system for several hours. A large helping of sugar causes the body to commandeer stored nutrients to metabolize (digest) the load of sugar dumped in it. Halloween, Christmas, Easter and Valentine's Day, when so many sweets are eaten, are hard on all, especially children. Doctors tell us that a day or two after these holidays their offices have the most cases of respiratory problems.

Sugar contributes to every known illness, from hyperactivity to arthritis, diabetes, cancer and chronic fatigue syndrome. The average person in the United States eats 125 pounds of this harmful, no-food food each year. There is an interesting side note about sugar. When tested, almost every person is found to be allergic to refined white table sugar. Almost no one is found to be allergic to raw sugar cane. And only a few test allergic to a raw crystallized sugar called succanat.

Pure, white table sugar is good for one thing: it is a powerful disinfectant. Poured into a fresh cut, burn, skin ulcer or a non-healing sore, it will, after a few applications, heal it, often without scarring. A number of physicians are discovering this. Others choose to follow profit-seeking pharmaceuticals and continue using drugs and medications, both slower to heal and causing side effects. The reason white table sugar (or raw, unstrained honey) is so very curative is that bacteria and virus cannot live in it. There is no oxygen. Dressed lightly with gauze, the sugar (or honey) treatment causes no sticking of the bandage, a decided advantage when treated again and dressed.

Around the turn of the century the Three Deadly Whites—sugar, flour and vegetable shortening (which includes margarine; it's white before it's artificially colored)— began to be produced. Suddenly cheap enough for everyone to buy because of mass production, they became the basis for the standard American diet. As a result, by 1910 heart disease was common. Vitamin E, essential for a healthy heart, had almost entirely disappeared from the diet. In 1890, before the Three Deadly Whites were generally and daily consumed, the average American got at least fifteen IU of vitamin E from his diet. But with the processing of hydrogenated vegetable oils, the use of white flour and the tremendous increase in the consumption of sugar, the American diet went from fifteen IU of vitamin E per person to 1.5, one-tenth of the former normal amount of vitamin E so necessary for healthy organs, especially the heart. White sugar, devoid of all vitamins and minerals, greatly contributes to the lowering of nutrients in the diet. White sugar contains no fiber. As though these nutrient disasters were not enough, eating the Three Deadly Whites displaces the eating of such natural foods as fresh vegetables, fruits, nuts, seeds and legumes with their enzymes, vitamins, minerals, fiber and oxygen.

The much-advocated "balanced diet" of the dietetic schools, supported by the medical profession and the food processing industry, held absolute sway from the 1920s to the 1970s. The food industry adopted the balanced diet concept totally, sending it through a willing, profit-sharing media to flood our country and indeed the whole world. The unquestioned "balanced diet" after World War II was so indelibly imprinted on our lifestyle that change could come about only through the great persistence of dedicated people interested in natural nutrition.

Not until recently did the world begin to heed the words of God's commandments and instructions about nutrition. Those utterances were rarely focused upon, pondered over, studied, or written about. Man took for granted the fact of eating food. To him, either the supply was amply provided in his allotted place and way of living or it was so scarce he struggled with life and limb to obtain enough for himself and his family. In the eyes of the general public, food was, and to a large extent still is food, and no matter what one eats he will somehow be sustained. Even today, with all the knowledge, research, clinical studies and evidence of nutrition playing a critical role in health and recovery, there are still doctors who say what a person eats has nothing to do with health and recovery from disease.

God, however, does not take lightly the matter of nourishment for the body. He knows it is all-important, so important He dealt with it first in the personal life of mankind. God calls the body "the temple of the soul." As such it must be recognized with utmost respect. It must be cared for constantly, regularly, consistently. The body is precious, one of a kind. It should function well at all times during the lifetime of its occupant. It is the only temple of the soul-spirit man will ever have on earth. It must last until God's purpose for that individual is completed and finished. For all this to take place, it must be nourished correctly.

That's why God gives us His commandment number one—the instruction on what to eat—in the first chapter of the first book of the Bible. To emphasize this instruction, He tells us in the last chapter of the last book of the Bible what we will eat in the reconstituted earth during the millennium: *"In the midst of the street of it [the throne of God], and on either side of the river, was there the tree of life, which bare twelve manner of fruits, and yielded her fruit every month: and the leaves of the tree were for the healing of the nations"* (Revelation 22:2).

But back to the dietetic dictum for eating, advocated from the 1920s to the 1970s. It is as follows:

- Proteins
- Starches
- Minerals
- Fruits and vegetables

What was wrong with this eating instruction from man who paid no heed to God's plan? Not a great deal, seventy years ago, except that much of it was cooked. Today it is a different story, with the overall answer being quite simple: most of those foods are processed, chemically treated with preservatives, sprayed, irradiated, canned, fried, over-cooked, altered and supplemented with artificial colors and flavor. As a result, they have been robbed of a multitude of nutrients and left with cooked, deficient starches (mostly from sugar and white flour), highly heated, indigestible, hard (hydrogenated) fats, a pauper's share of fiber and a critical dearth of minerals.

In many other ways those foods are even further reduced in nutritional value. After the trip home from the supermarket, many foods, such as fresh vegetables, are heated or cooked in the microwave, a tragic heating process that totally alters amino acids, among other things. (Microwaves are food destroyers.) In addition to a lack of minerals in plants around the world because of soils impoverished from over cultivation, there is extra spraying to "protect" the product from insect infestation, spoilage and rancidity. By law, foods imported from other countries into the United States have to be sprayed. Even the time lapse between farm and market contributes to nutrient loss through oxidation.

With all this happening to foods, one wonders how man ever avoids diseases. We also wonder how there can be any sort of "balanced diet" of greatly altered, fractionated, devitalized, killed, partially destroyed, chemicalized and overcooked food. In other words, how can junk foods ever provide a balanced diet? No intelligent, serious-minded person is foolish enough to think even for a minute that such a thing is possible. Yet many actually live on junk food. Most people do not want to be bothered with exposure to such a sobering truth. They don't want their own little worlds disturbed. They don't wish to take responsibility for their own health. As a result, they are unhealthy and sick.

A few examples of such untreated foods as fresh vegetables will readily show how shocking these stark truths can be. Let's start with serving one medium, sixty-five–gram, raw carrot, which is roughly equivalent to three cooked carrots of equal size. The raw carrot is a complete food, although the nutrients are not in proportion to what the body requires over a period of time. The carrot has vitamins, minerals, bulk (fiber), starch, fruit sugar, water, protein, enzymes, oxygen and micro-nutrients. This one medium, sixty-five–gram carrot will have twenty-eight calories.

Three medium-sized carrots cooked to the tenderness of canned or restaurant carrots, having lost some of their calories in the cooking water, will still contain more than twice the calories of the raw carrot. They will also have lost much of their natural water, most of their vitamins, some of their minerals and micro-nutrients (through leaching into the cooking water), and their oxygen. All of their enzymes, so necessary for good digestion and assimilation, are killed. One medium-sized raw carrot is considered a vegetable serving, as are three medium-sized, cooked carrots, usually considered of equal nutrition. The eater of the raw carrot has complete nutrition with only twenty-eight calories. The eater of the cooked carrots has incomplete and deficient nutrition, yet with two to three times the calories (sixty to eighty) that the single, whole-nutrition raw carrot has.

This cooked food principle, extended across the whole spectrum of cooked food, gives part of the answer for people being overfed and undernourished. It accounts for part of the basis of weight gain. By eating all natural, mostly raw fruits, vegetables, seeds (sprouted), nuts (soaked), grains (germinated) and budded legumes soaked overnight for minimum budding, the body is satisfied without being overfed. By the time a person is overweight, his health problems have had a good start, although that fact may not yet be noticed and recognized or admitted. But by the time a person is obese, he suffers minor to major health problems, many of which are life threatening. Craving for sweets or highly processed, fractionated foods ceases as the body becomes cleansed and sufficient chromium, an essential mineral, is obtained from the diet or from a chromium supplement. Overeating is rarely a problem when a cleansed body gets only natural foods. It is nearly impossible to overeat of raw, bulky foods. Cooked, processed, concentrated, impacted foods filling the stomach invariably mean eating more calories than the body can burn for heat and energy. Those unburned calories are converted by an already overworked liver to fat cells in the body, fat that is much easier for most people to put on than take off. Continuing in this sort of eating style steadily leads from normal weight to *over*weight, then to obesity.

Is it any wonder? First, we have not eaten the *all-natural* way God initially told us to eat. Second, we have too often overindulged our appetites and overeaten. Third, we have consistently disregarded the welfare of our bodies, abusing it even further with poisons and addictive beverages and drinks. We have grossly ignored the care and feeding of the only body we'll ever have here on earth.

The Scriptures leave no doubt about what God considers *right* foods. By deduction we arrive at the truth about *wrong* foods. They are all the cooked and processed foods which the majority of the people in the developed nations of the world eat. Is that so bad? Physically, yes.

Morally, no, it is not so bad because God in His permissive will permits the eating of them without condemnation. Under the New Testament covenant, eating them is no sin. However, we eat them at great risk. We eat them because it is what the world does and we are in the world. We tend to follow what the world does. Unfortunately, those foods for many are all that are available. They do help people to survive. They do maintain and sustain a low-performance life. They just do not give health. They do not provide for prevention or maximum energy and mental, emotional, physical and spiritual performance. For these reasons they are considered *wrong*.

From wrong eating we suffer deficiencies more and more. One of these deficiencies is the trace mineral chromium, responsible for the metabolism of sugars. Without adequate chromium a person craves sweets and starches, especially starches made of white flour, such as pastas, bread, rolls, puddings, cakes, cookies and gravies. Coupled with an improved diet, chromium can lessen the craving for these things and help the body metabolize sugars and lose weight, especially if exercise is part of the program.

Remember! God told us what to eat while on this earth in the first chapter of the first book of the Bible. I quote it again because it is all-important: *". . . Behold, I have given you every herb bearing seed, which is upon the face of all the earth, and every tree, in the which is the fruit of a tree yielding seed; to you it shall be for [food]"* (Genesis 1:29). Then in the last chapter of the last book of the Bible, He told us what we will eat during the Millennium on the renewed earth. I quote it again: *"In the midst of the street of it [the holy city of Jerusalem], and on either side of the river, was there the tree of life, which bare twelve manner of fruits, and yielded her fruit every month: and the leaves of the tree were for the healing of the nations"* (Revelation 22:2).

Doesn't it go without saying that God wanted and still wants us to eat living, oxygenated, raw foods, the best He has to offer to keep our bodies in the best condition possible? By so doing, we can maintain, even in an imperfect world, the temple of our souls in excellent health, high activity, and maximum mental and emotional function.

Chapter Seven

THE DRASTIC RESULTS OF MISSING THE COMMANDMENT

The fascinating news is that God's way works, because He planned all creation for and around man. He did not make man, His ultimate creation, to accommodate or to conform to the universe. For instance, He assured us the Sabbath was for man, not man for the Sabbath. So it was with the plants in the Garden of Eden. All those wonderful fruit trees were of course very beautiful, certainly an aesthetic blessing. They were also for man's physical needs, providing shade and food. Thus, trees with their fruits and seeds supplied most of the amenities necessary for living—nourishment, enjoyment, protection, well-being, satisfaction and perfect health.

God also gave man the privilege of choice. However, having provided so amply for His creation's needs, He made one reservation about choices. He had His reason for doing so. He told Adam and Eve not to eat the fruits of the tree of knowledge. But Eve, pleased with Eden, her new home

51

with its great beauty and wonder, was open to all it had to offer. In fact, being young and inexperienced, she could also have been a bit naive. Intrigued by Satan's beguiling words, she said, "We may eat fruit from the trees in the garden." Then, as an afterthought, she added, "But God did say, 'You must not eat fruit from the tree that is in the middle of the garden, and you must not touch it, or you will die!'"

"You will not surely die," the serpent assured her. "For God knows that when you eat of it your eyes will be opened and you will be like God, knowing good and evil."

No match at the time for the subtle cunning of Satan, Eve was persuaded to eat of the forbidden fruit and to give some to her husband. God straightway cursed her tempter, then pronounced these awesome words to Adam and his wife: ". . . You will eat the plants of the field." (See Genesis 3:1–18.)

The plants of the field were second best, not at all the luscious, perfect fruits of the Garden. In addition to fruits, plants of the field included anything edible that grows in fields—roots, pods, bark, leaves, seeds and grains. Although we know that man's life after sinning could no longer last forever as planned, we also know that he did live, after the Fall, nine-hundred-plus years on such fare, and in good health.

Man was created—and still is—a fruit eater (a frugavore). He has biting teeth to cut into crisp fruits, such as apples. However, his food outside the Garden included hard roots and tough barks, which his teeth could handle. His grinding teeth could crush seeds, grains and the roughest, toughest of natural, edible fibers. The acid of his stomach, one tenth as strong as that of meat-eating animals, was just right for the easily digested fruit and vegetable proteins of his raw foods. And his intestines, three times longer than a carnivore's, provided for plenty of peristaltic (squeezing) action to extract (digest) the nutrients from the fiber for efficient assimilation and absorption into his bloodstream, to be carried to all the cells of his body.

That body was "fearfully and wondrously made." (See Psalm 139:14.) And the food of the earth was just right to nourish it optimally. The Garden of Eden that Adam and Eve had to leave grew all manner of fruits and edible plants. In the first chapter of Genesis, God told about the food growing not only in the Garden, but over all the earth. *"And the earth brought forth grass, and herb yielding seed after his kind, and the tree yielding fruit, whose seed was in itself, after his kind: and God saw that it was good"* (Genesis 1:12).

That's what the early people ate just as God had commanded. On that diet they lived their long lifespan.

In the initial plan, Adam and Eve were to enjoy perfect health in the Garden of Eden where vegetation abounded— all the food they needed, ready to eat. There was no sickness, no death.

Health without blemish and perfect contentment were the design for them. *". . . Everything that has the breath of life in it—I give every green plant for food"* (Genesis 1:30, NIV).

When temptation came, curiosity and desire to taste the fruit took over and Adam and Eve yielded to that temptation. How interesting to observe that both God's first commandment and man's first sin had to do with food. Because of this sin of disobedience, the first couple became vulnerable to both sickness and death.

Sent forth from Eden, they were made to realize that man would from that time on have to till the ground. *". . .*

Cursed is the ground because of you; through painful toil you will eat of it all the days of your life. It will produce thorns and thistles for you, and you will eat the plants of the field. By the sweat of your brow you will eat your food until you return to the ground" (Genesis 3:17–19, NIV). We now understand how man, for ten generations of eating fruits, vegetables, seeds and nuts lived so many years. We also understand why, since then, by deliberately turning away from God's first commandment, man's health has steadily gone downhill. At the rate it's going, two in every three people will have some form of cancer in his lifetime by the year 2000, plus any number of other serious diseases. The greatest single cause for this state of physical welfare is our disobedience to God's commandment regarding eating. The lifespan before the Flood:

- Adam   930 years
- Seth   912 years
- Enos   905 years
- Cain   910 years
- Methuselah 969 years
- Lamech   777 years
- Noah   950 years

This averages out to a 912-year lifespan.

For ten generations after the Flood:

- Noah   950 years
- Shem   600 years
- Arphaxad   438 years
- Salah   433 years
- Eber   464 years

- Peleg   239 years
- Ren   239 years
- Serug   230 years
- Mahor   206 years
- Abraham 175 years

This averages out to a 336-year lifespan.

We here review two important facts and add a third and fourth that undoubtedly contributed to the shortening of the lifespan after the Flood.

The *first* was the lowered oxygen content in the air due to the reduced air pressure when the sea level settled three miles higher than where man had previously lived.

The *second* was lowered oxygen, which resulted in disease: the appearance of bacteria, viruses, molds, amoebae and decay.

The *third* was the drastic change in diet, from plants to animal flesh and some cooked plants.

The *fourth* was the disappearance of the vapor canopy that completely surrounded the earth until the Flood. This vapor had filtered out the sun's ultraviolet rays. Man, shielded from these harmful rays and taking in plenty of oxygen and complete, living foods, had been so protected that his body not only lived for many centuries, it was able to use all of his wonderful mind. Scientists tell us that today we use less than ten percent of our brains.

Since food is a very important reason for lowered lifespan (over which we have considerable control), let's see just what we can do about our consumption of it.

The digestion of food requires the expenditure of energy. Meat and cooked foods take more than three times the energy to be digested than a meal of living fruits and vegetables. This translates into more energy being available for activities. Most of us would welcome feeling great and having more energy. That is what we get when we eat all-natural, mostly raw foods.

We are assured that life is in the blood. *"Only be sure that thou eat not the blood: for the blood is the life; and thou mayest not eat the life with the flesh"* (Deuteronomy 12:23). When that blood is pure, the body is pure. Clean. Free of disease. Healthy. The brain and nervous system function well.

Obeying the natural laws laid down for man carries the rich reward not only of health but also of longevity. Moses is a wonderful example. In all his 120 years he obeyed God's laws and experienced no disease during his long lifetime. His eyesight never failed, his hearing remained acute, his hair stayed free from gray, and his strength never lessened. He died a natural death. His way of eating pleased God. It allowed him to live out the healthy lifespan allotted him. He had beautifully fulfilled his purpose on Earth.

What is the key to receiving such blessings? Obeying God. Following His commandments. It means dedication to please Him, to glorify Him, to serve Him. In a word, we eat to please Him because He expects us to take care of our bodies, His temple. God says to glorify Him in our bodies: *"For ye are bought with a price: therefore glorify God in your body, and in your spirit, which are God's"* (I Corinthians 6:20).

One of our greatest responsibilities is to take care of our body, to feed it correctly. We are the stewards of all we have and should not misuse or abuse that responsibility, that commission. *". . . Know ye not that ye are the temple of God, and that the Spirit of God dwelleth in you?"* (I Corinthians 3:16).

Chapter Eight

DOES DEAD FOOD
LEAD TO ADDICTION?

Dead foods and food addictions are not usually discussed in the same breath. However, they might well be since dead foods can actually cause food addiction.

So what is dead food? No, it's not a deceased animal's carcass. The dead food we are talking about is cooked and/or processed food. Heat, as has been said, kills. Destroys. It does all these things to living vegetables, fruits, seeds, nuts and sprouts. Generally speaking, 50 percent of the nutrition in foods, when cooked, is destroyed, wasted, broken down. A sprig of cooked spinach, if steamed only a few minutes, is little more than a carcass because most of its nutrients have been destroyed except its fiber. Its color is dulled and it is limp. Could you get a cow to eat it? When the sprig of cooked spinach is laid beside a sprig of uncooked spinach which is bright green, crisp, beautiful and full of life, one can see which sprig will give more life.

Food addiction, simply explained, is a pronounced craving for a certain food or foods. A so-called chocoholic is a prime example of a person troubled with food addiction. Sugar is the large part of the addiction. This abnormal craving for chocolate may cause him to frequently binge on that rich, tasty sweet. Or the craving might be whole wheat bread, as I had for several years until it was revealed that wheat was, next to sugar, my worst enemy. It caused me so great a lowering of energy, as did sugar, that I could not work. At times I could scarcely walk across the room or talk, so intense was the fatigue. My therapist called it severe addiction associated with allergy to wheat.

Or the addiction might be to junk foods. Indeed, many people are addicted to them—fried foods, hamburgers, burritos, hot dogs, pizza, cokes, fruit drinks, coffee (espresso, mocha, latté, etc.) ice cream, many kinds of commercial cookies, candies, chili dogs, white flour, pork, spaghetti, macaroni, and so on. These are all dead foods, cooked, fractionated, processed. People who frequently eat these foods often become addicted to them.

By contrast, live, raw foods are rarely found to be addictive. They are whole foods. Because they are whole they are full of natural nutrients. Because they have all those nutrients they are satisfying. Because they satisfy they do not leave the body severely craving for more and more. Without craving, the eater rarely becomes addicted. Nor is the temptation there to overeat, because the body is well nourished and satisfied without being stuffed.

When we eat dead foods we are so undernourished that the body often demands something more because of its need for that missing something to maintain its normal function.

There are many non-foods—ice cream made with artificial ingredients, whipped cream substitute, olestra, eggless, non-fat mayonnaise, processed cake frosting, etc.—which satisfy our sense of taste but only deceive us. We think they are wonderful because they are "delicious, inexpensive and non-fattening," according to the food processor. Anything that tastes so good, in the opinion of nearly everyone, must be good for us. Yet the opposite is often true. The satisfaction we receive from our taste or craving for foods makes us look toward the same foods for the next meal and the next and the one after that until we no longer are able to make good choices. Our "appestat" has broken down. Our bodies and senses have become addicted to the deficient and false foods we became accustomed to eating.

The most addictive foods are cooked foods. The advertising of a "good, hot meal" has universal appeal. We have been raised mainly on "good, hot" cooked foods. We live on cooked foods. It's the way of the world.

When we eat dead food, we may eventually reap its reward: degenerative disease. It may take years but it will come. For good health, reasonable longevity, and prevention, the body must have all the nutrients plus the life force in the foods it consumes. Processed, cooked, chemically enhanced foods only keep us going at a subnormal pace. They do not give health. Little by little they leave the body so depleted and undernourished that it is actually crippled because of malnutrition. Consequently, overeating of the very foods that cause the problem perpetuates the condition. The poor, meager diet fails to maintain the body's ability to function, to give it energy and sufficient strength and a good immune system. This failure to maintain allows the door to degeneration to open. As with a chain, it is the weakest link that fails first. So too with the body. Disease will attack the area most weakened by lack of nourishment. For instance, that weakest place, area or organ may be the eyes. According to reports by doctors who are aware of nutrition as a prime factor in the treatment and prevention of disease, most eye problems start with a deficiency of vitamins C, A and B2, in that order, followed by a lack of all the B vitamins. Or the weakest link may be joints where arthritis sets in. This increasing problem usually starts with a deficiency of magnesium, the main mineral necessary for calcium to be properly metabolized instead of accumulating in soft tissues and/or being deposited on the joints. Magnesium is found in dark green leafy vegetables, whole grains, seeds and nuts. A plethora of poverty-stricken white foods—sugar, flour, processed fats and oils, white rice, white pastas, pasteurized, homogenized milk, and too much commercially grown and processed meat—are among the main causes of arthritis. They overload the system, impacting the bowel and lowering the immune system. They cause the body to struggle to compensate any way it can for the lack of nutrition.

Such eating habits place a tremendous burden on the kidneys and the colon, among other organs and systems. The colon receives the waste from wrong foods, from undigested nutrients that putrefy in the small intestines. It is our garbage dump where degenerative disease gets it start. Plainly, we are instructed to eat fresh, living foods that readily digest and quickly pass down, keeping our system clean and functioning at peak performance. We are told not to defile our bodies. If we do, they will be subject to premature destructive forces. To eat wrong is slow suicide.

Healing ministries are precious, but perhaps more precious is a healthy body. If it functions optimally, it is well and needs no healing. There are certain peoples on the earth who have none of the ills of modern man. The Hunzas of the Himalayan Mountains are such a group. They have no problems with being overweight, no heart disease, no eye or digestion problems, no cancer or birth defects to speak of. They live on an all-natural, mostly uncooked diet with very little meat. By contrast, in our highly *civilized* and scientifically oriented society, where we eat our refined, technologically produced foods, we rarely find a totally healthy person, young or old. Disease is that rampant and out of control.

How can we expect God to bless the food we eat when it is so unlike what He has given us to nourish ourselves? The majority of God's "faithful" do not eat the foods He ordained in the Bible. They ignore the Scriptures. They regularly eat pork and shellfish, "unclean meats," at great risk to their health. They have fallen into gluttony because they have abused their bodies. Their appetites, distorted by indulgence in wrong foods over a period of time, cannot be relied upon, and they frequently overeat. The wild creatures can depend on their keen sense of smell to tell them what not to eat. Man's senses are so dulled by cooked and processed foods, chemicals and pollution in the air and in the water that he cannot rely on them to protect himself from foods that are wrong for him. We have been led to believe that modern man has permanently lost much of his senses, particularity the sense of smell. However, this is untrue. After a water fast (at least a week for most of us), the acuteness of the senses—smell, taste, sight, hearing and touch—usually returns. After my first nine-day fast of just pure water and a few pinches of pure sea salt daily to keep me from dehydrating and losing energy, I was amazed at how acute each of my senses was.

61

Just like wild animals, I could "sense" what was right for my body in the correct amount. We fall into the habit of gluttony because we often cannot sense when we've had enough until we have had too much.

How incredible this all is when we consider the thousands upon thousands today teaching the Bible, yet overlooking this all-important message on feeding the temple of the soul, the body.

Increasingly, there is emphasis on healing among believers. But where is the emphasis on teaching about foods, about eating, about obeying God's instructions on the sustenance and care of the body?

The Apostle Paul admonishes us to be temperate in all things. Everyone knows that overeating can lead to overweight, obesity and disease when the diet is saturated with addictive sweets made with white flour and sugar. Such foods in Biblical times were indulged in only on special occasions, like weddings, holy days, feast days and birthdays. All were times for celebration and rejoicing. Such sweet foods were never meant to be eaten every day and surely not to be taken as a full meal. Breakfasts today are frequently filled with sugar—the non-food—devoid of any nutrition whatsoever except naked calories. (There are doctors who classify white sugar as a drug because it is addictive.) Prepared and processed foods are often loaded with sugar and/or fructose (corn syrup), which rob the body of stored nutrients in order to be metabolized. Or they are loaded with artificial sweeteners such as aspartame, which are as harmful as sugar. Some people say they can be even more harmful.

Three commonly used artificial sweeteners are aspartame, saccharin, and sorbitol. Aspartame, widely used in soft drinks, desserts, and wherever sugar is used, is especially harmful since it causes, among many other problems, brain alteration, nerve, eye and seizure problems, headaches, and eventually weight gain instead of weight loss, a major reason it is touted. The Center for Disease Control in Atlanta has recorded more complaints caused by aspartame than by any other substance.

For a time the FDA would not allow stevia, a natural sweetener, to be imported as a food. The leaf of the stevia plant is many times sweeter than sugar, strengthens instead of harms the adrenal glands, is pleasant to taste, and in its dry, powdered leaf form has great shelf life. It can now be bought as powdered leaf or in liquid concentrate form at health food stores where it was formerly sold as a cosmetic.

We must remember that at the beginning of the twentieth century, food processing started coming into general use. White flour, sugar, shortening and margarine started appearing on the tables of most households. The age of advertisement and propaganda came into being. Slogans and messages urged the public to buy whatever tasted good. This quickly helped lead people to indulge in all sorts of foods that catered to their growing addiction to sweets, fats and alcohol. Small wonder that today, near the end of the twentieth century, 60 percent of the population is overweight and 34 percent is obese, largely because of white flour and white sugar. Nearly fifty percent of the children are overweight. Two generations ago a chubby child was rare, and a "plump, fleshy" adult was the exception to the rule of normal weight.

We cry out to God to heal us, to make us well, to protect us from sickness, yet we continue to bring malaise down upon ourselves by lack of discipline in eating, by our wants and desires for what tastes good. It makes one wonder about what we say we want and what we do to achieve our wants. We don't do this deliberately. We do it because we fail to recognize the divine laws on how to eat and maintain our health. We err by default. What follows for many of us is a continuation of the way of eating that made us sick in the first place. As long as most of us eat according to our compulsive appetites, health statistics will continue to be increasingly frightening.

Sadly, many Christians, including pastors, ministers, counselors and leaders in church outreaches, consume a lot of junk food. They love to make light of it and even to joke about their failures and indulgences. The majority of their congregations fail to be the example of living God's way. In essence, they are rejecting God's ordained foods and His laws. Perhaps they feel these Scriptures do not apply to them or those they guide through the realm of spiritual life. Like people in general, pastors and their flocks accept the "unquestioned fact" that it is entirely normal for men and women to get sick with a number of diseases as they grow older, then die. What a contrast to what is taught in the Bible, and the examples given therein.

Just as God allows sickness and disease to come upon people of loose character, so He allows sickness and disease to come upon those of good moral character when His guidelines for proper eating habits are ignored and not followed. Believers and non-believers alike are accustomed to eating everything sold in supermarkets, mini-marts and restaurants, and all get sick in the same way.

Chapter Nine

CAN DISEASE BE CONQUERED?

We *can* conquer disease. To do so we must break with present day customs and deal with basic, traditional foods. Change is difficult for most people. But change can be challenge, adventure, new worlds to conquer if we approach it with the freshness of anticipation and new vision, with originality and faith to please God.

Daily we read and hear about the bad side effects of prescription drugs. The Physicians Desk Reference (PDR) verifies this flood of information. And daily we watch the statistics on dreaded degenerative disease go up, and the statistics on iatrogenic disease—drug/hospital/doctor-induced sickness and death—go right up with them.

In our enlightened age, how can this be? Our scientists can put men on the moon, a library of information on a micro-chip. Our physicians can transplant a living heart to give a terminal patient a normal lifespan. Our mechanical and electronic engineers can send masses of people and tons of cargo through the air at only a little less than the speed of sound. Why can we do so little with our health statistics? For instance, take glaucoma and macular degeneration, the greatest causes of blindness. The disease of glaucoma is almost epidemic, and the resulting blindness is increasing. One enterprising medical journalist took it upon himself to research the problem. He found that most physicians diagnose glaucoma based only on eye fluid pressure readings and blame the development of the disease on this single factor. Yet after a century of hypotensive therapy for the optic atrophy called glaucoma, there is evidence enough to make one question how effective it is. In fact, researchers in the field have been led to ask whether the disease itself is any more detrimental than the treatment.

At the same time, there are at least two natural therapies available by a number of dedicated people who have brought about remission of this dreaded problem. There is also a woman ophthalmologist who is having great success in teaching people how to help themselves through mostly natural means. But because these modalities have not been proven by double blind studies, they are little known and rarely written about. Yet the therapies are natural, without side effects. There is nothing to be lost if they do not bring about remission. However, in many cases they joyously conquer the eye problem.

Then there is cancer. Studies have been made of hundreds of cancer cases over a period of many years. These studies reveal that cancer surgery patients who submit to radiation and/or chemotherapy live approximately three and a half years after treatment. Cancer surgery patients who refuse those debilitating, cell-destroying treatments live approximately twelve and a half years, roughly four times longer. And without the devastating suffering of the "therapy."

Are we so blinded, so intimidated, so impressed by what we think is the infallibility of science? The awesome "advances" of the medical community? The overwhelming multiplicity of allopathic remedies and resources? Are the majority of us so affected, so panicked by it all, that we flock to the offices of conventional doctors, fill hospitals and clinics with our problems, demand tests and x-rays and scans and diagnoses of specialists of every kind?

How many people have you heard say this: "I've been to many doctors, specialists and therapists and I'm no better"?

At such a time we frequently find ourselves, in our own case, at our wits' end, partially non-functional. What have we done, or are doing, wrong? Surely, with all the supplements and natural remedies and herbals out there something can be found to give us hope: vitamins, minerals, amino acids; strange new miracle substances with abbreviated, long names like coenzyme Q10, or pycnogenol, or DHEA, or condroitan sulphate; commonly known foods that are being touted as near cure-alls, like cayenne pepper, garlic and the juice of plain old cabbage.

Our first thought is what we can take to help us. Yet the first thing to do is to take out—delete, avoid, eliminate—processed foods and synthetic supplements. Take the bad food out of our diets. Then carry on with basic, natural foods, herbal teas and natural supplements. In other words, we go back and start at the beginning.

"In the beginning" there were no processed foods.
We take out all processed foods.
There were no fractionated grains, i.e. white flour.
We take out white flour and white rice.

There were no synthetic, artificial foods. *We take out all such things as non-dairy creamers and artificial whipped cream, butter substitutes such as margarine, no matter how carefully whipped, colored and flavored, egg beater products, ice creams and synthetic, harmful oils.* There were none of these originally. *We take out all preservatives, additives, artificial colorings and flavors.* None of these existed before the steady, devastating breakdown of health in the twentieth century.

We take out all refined sugar, a product that is a non-food food, so foreign to the body that it causes nothing but lowered health, hyperactivity, lessened energy, a shut-down immune system and a shortened lifespan. And we take out chemically aged cheese and synthetic vinegars. The list goes on.

What is left to eat, you ask? Surprisingly, a great deal— all delicious, colorful, healthful and satisfying: seeds, nuts, grains, legumes, fruits and vegetables, honey, carob and a host of delightful herbs and spices for flavor. And there are delicate, mild and pleasant teas.

In my long experience of eating, teaching, advocating, writing about and demonstrating living (raw) foods, I have never heard one person who has truly adopted the all-natural way of eating speak negatively of this lifestyle. He or she always says, "I feel so much better"; or "I have such good energy"; or "My problems improved"; "My health troubles went away"; "I enjoy the great tastes and flavors of natural foods"; "My mind is clear."

Though they are a minority, these people make up a larger segment of health-conscious people every year. And their numbers are increasing. They are the joyous enlightened ones. The rest of the people are tossed about in a churning, man-polluted sea, only to be eventually swept asunder by the rising tide of disease, fail-related health, and accident; or they are caught in the undertow of end-time pestilence and plague, super stress, emotional breakdown and depression.

Many voices have sounded the alarm and many more have joined the chorus to proclaim the saving news. But to go with the news means change. In the eyes of many it means going back to the archaic. It means throwing out and stopping the "progress" of the last century.

Unfortunately, to many all this is quackery, old wives' tales, rubbish and nutritional nonsense. Besides, who's to say all this is true? Where's the proof?

We have only to turn to the Bible. Try it before you condemn the whole idea. God provided for all our needs and it is recorded there: everything to eat, not only for our health and very sustenance, but for our joy and pleasure, our feasting and festivities. For our health maintenance there are vegetables, and for our healing, pleasant herbs and "bitter" herbs. (The bitterness in herbs is a white crystalline substance that becomes oxygen in the body, oxygen being the blood purifier, the greatest healing element.)

Many cultures around the world have had their traditional healing herbs. In recent years medical science has been turning back to and rediscovering many of these plants. As a matter of fact, there have been and still are international meetings on herbs of the world and their place in the pharmacopoeia of remedies for all diseases. Another natural healing modality is homeopathy, an effective, proven medical practice that has been around since the 1820s.

Why should we continue to go our own destructive way until we are ill, desperate or hopeless? Eating the unnatural way—overeating, taking in our fill of artificial, carcinogenic foods and intoxicating drinks—takes us down the path to degenerated health in body and in mind. It is inevitable. It is death by disease, slow, depressing and painful to the end. We wouldn't think of feeding our pet deer or parakeet or even our dog doughnuts and coffee, cooked vegetables, hot dogs and ice cream, coke, beer and pretzels. They would all sicken and die long before their allotted time. Yet that's exactly what is happening to us as a nation. Instead of our assigned one hundred and twenty years, we live into our early, predicted seventies if we are lucky, and even that precious time is usually fraught with pain and problems.

Prevention is the answer. An optimal diet for parents before conception and for pregnant women is one that contains minerals, vitamins, enzymes and oxygen, all of which are found in fruits, nuts, seeds, vegetables and naturally produced animal products. Much is appearing in the news media, in journals and magazines, on television and the radio about such nutrients as folic acid for prevention of birth defects; magnesium and B6 for avoiding early-on nausea and the critical development of the mandibular (jawbone joint), the teeth and the brain; zinc for sexual organ development; and on and on.

Clearly the answer is wholesome, natural nutrition before conception, through pregnancy and birth, childhood and adulthood, to old age and the grave. It is vital, necessary, or we die sickly and before our time. Surely it is not so hard to do, to avoid the wasted and eat the wholesome in order to enjoy the radiant energy of a well-functioning body, free of disease.

Chapter Ten

GREAT FOODS
OF THE BIBLE

In the Scriptures we are given the types and names of the many foods God provided for us. Although they are mentioned several times throughout the Bible, some are especially ignored or held in question or even opposed by present day believers of the Bible.

A case in point would be that of butter. Butter of kine (cows), is referred to eleven times in the Bible, each time favorably. We first read about it in Genesis. Abraham was sitting in the door of his tent when the three travelers (the Lord and two angels) appeared. After greeting them and washing their feet, as was the custom, Abraham set before them bread, a freshly dressed calf, milk and butter. *"And he took butter, and milk, and the calf which he [the young servant] had dressed, and set it before them; and he stood by them under the tree, and they did eat"* (Genesis 18:8). There is no mention of cooking the calf meat. The original Hebrew text says only, "which he had dressed." Some versions of the text infer that it was cooked, some say it was roasted. The servant simply dressed it and Abraham set it before the three, along with the bread, milk and butter. (Dressing an animal for eating is another way of saying butchered.)

Incredibly, butter began to fall out of favor in the early 1920s just as margarine was becoming universally popular. A powerful food industry put out such extensive propaganda that every man, woman and child knew about margarine. Every newspaper, magazine and radio carried ads for it. Samples were given out in grocery stores. It was presented as having a better taste, being fresher and not as fattening, not as perishable and yet costing much less than butter. As the years went by and people became more health conscious, a rumor circulated countrywide that butter was unhealthy; that it was bad for the heart; that it contributed to high blood pressure; that it was difficult to digest and caused weight problems. Strangely, many doctors joined the margarine bandwagon to extol its "superior" quality as a fat food and to condemn butter because of its content of hard fat, which they maintained was a threat to the heart.

A case of "true lies" had been established. In a few years, the polyunsaturated fat content of margarine was big news. Its cholesterol-free quality was extolled to those who wanted to *cut the risk* of heart disease. The medical profession fell in line with this now-prevalent attitude of margarine being the *healthy choice.* Then with the continued rise in heart disease and the increase in deaths that inevitably followed, most doctors ordered the commercial polyunsaturated margarine for their patients.

All during this time there were the voices of scientists and researchers who knew that margarine, processed vegetables oils and shortening were hydrogenated and loaded with chemicals—solvents, bleach, artificial color and artificial flavor. Heated to high temperatures, they should not be eaten at all. They actually cause or contribute to the very problems they are said to alleviate. It is beyond comprehension that decades passed before the magnitude of the deception was made known and the real story began to filter down to the public.

All the while, the truth lay firmly, quietly, majestically in the *Word.* A few perceptive individuals, schooled in nutrition, began to reveal the correct ways to eat in order for nutrients to be metabolized. Actually, these truths were already in print right under our very noses. The Bible rings forth with a multitude of direct and indirect references to how people should behave in the area of eating. And, once again, many of these nutrition-minded people began to be looked upon in a less than favorable light. Who wants to hear what a few "extremists" have to say, especially when what they say will affect the "modern" way we live and why we live the way we do? But time reveals truths, even to the most stubborn of us all.

In the last few years some wonderfully useful facts have surfaced as a result of the works, study, and experience of an impressive number of scientists, physicians, therapists and nutritionists in our country and in many others around the world.

It has been discovered that the body needs and utilizes a small amount of hard fat, the kind that is found in butter. Without this natural hard fat, people stand a greater risk of developing cancer. Many cancer patients have eaten no natural hard fat for years.

It is also widely known and recognized that the processing of polyunsaturated, commercial vegetables oils, shortenings and margarine has turned the essential sis-linolenic acid to indigestible, unusable trans-linolenic acid, the exact opposite of sis-linolenic. In the same way, sis-linoleic acid, also an essential oil, is transformed to unusable trans-linoleic acid. Trans-linolenic and trans-linoleic acids, as these oils are known, cause sticky plaque to form on the walls of the arteries. The bad kind of cholesterol—LDL—and fats such as the broken-down cream molecule of homogenized milk, clings to and collects on this sticky plaque and clogs the blood vessels. Some physicians consider the sticky plaque to be the greatest problem of the arteries.

Back to the good—HDL—cholesterol. The body makes cholesterol from the starches we eat. Bad cholesterol—LDL—is made from bad carbohydrates like white flour products, white sugar and to a lesser degree, white rice. The good cholesterol is made from cooked and raw root vegetables (starches) and whole grain foods, seeds and nuts, honey, maple syrup, molasses and so on, all in moderation.

Only in the past few years has such information broken through to the general public. Some doctors are beginning to take notice of these findings of research, but the process is slow. "Doctors can be slow learners," says my family physician.

It appears that butter is coming back into favor, as the information on margarine is putting itself more and more in the background. Yet butter has always had God's sanction. He led Jacob about, lovingly looking after him, making him ride on the high places, eating the increase of the fields. *"... And he made him to suck honey out of the rock ... butter of kine, and milk..."* (Deuteronomy 32: 13–14).

To honor David and celebrate his outdoing the enemy on the other side of the Jordan, the people of Mahanaim

took *". . . Honey, and butter, and sheep, and cheese of kine"*
to the conquering army. (See II Samuel 17:29.)

In the words of Isaiah, butter is among the wonderful
promises. Speaking of the coming birth and life of the
Messiah, he wrote: *"Butter and honey shall he eat, that he
may know to refuse the evil and choose the good"* (Isaiah
7:15). The eating of a little butter soothes the body and
calms the mind. It makes for mental balance. It's satisfying
effect removes unnatural cravings and urges to overeat. In
a continuing prophecy, Isaiah, speaking of the remnant of
God's believers after the Assyrian captivity, assures them
of an abundance and the very choicest of foods: *". . . For
butter and honey shall everyone eat that is left in the land"*
(Isaiah 7:22).

The problem with butter, as with any extra good food,
is overindulgence in it. Eating too much of this recommended special delicacy is like eating too much of anything
else: it can be harmful. All health practitioners are in agree-
ment on this point, including doctors. Butter consumption
should not exceed one tablespoon (three patties) per day
for a large person, and two teaspoons (two patties) for children and an average to small-sized person. So we can continue to eat butter and enjoy it, for it stands high on God's
list of foods. And let us remember the Apostle Paul's words:
*"And every man that striveth for the mastery is temperate
in all things"* (I Corinthians 9:25).

Olive oil is another food that has gone up and down in
reputation in the past one hundred years. As commercially
processed oils filled the market shelves, olive oil fell into
disfavor. Some said the flavor of the oil was too overpower-
ing when compared to the more delicate (tasteless, altered,
processed) commercial oils. They also said the hard fat content of olive oil was not good for us.

Once again, the lobbying power of large food processors succeeded in instilling in the consumer the message that the clear, clean-looking oil in the brightly labeled bottles was far superior to anything nature had to offer. The housewife was soon brainwashed into believing she had to have an odorless, colorless, sedimentless, tasteless oil that could sit out of the refrigerator and not go stale. The interesting fact is that no insect or animal will touch it, much less eat it. Not only is there little or no food value in it, but it is also loaded with harmful chemicals. Man is the only creature that will eat hydrogenated oils and margarine.

Meanwhile, the so-called diehards who continued to use butter also realized that olive oil in its most natural state is far better for the body than the mass-produced, highly touted oils that sit on the supermarket shelves. Olive oil has finally regained its place among fine natural foods. God had provided mankind with this stable food, and man in America at long last has recognized it. Like butter, olive oil contains some hard fat. Unlike butter, olive oil is known for its remarkable stability. Its shelf life is superior to that of most natural oils. It keeps well out of refrigeration for weeks, even months. *It also contains the two essential oils— linoleic and linolenic acid.* Try dipping bread in it as the Italians do. It's delicious! Especially with whole grain breads.

Grapes appear throughout the Bible. Not only were they an integral part of the diet of man from the beginning, but they figure in the symbolism of poetry and song. Food analysts of the last two or three decades have found many nutrients in grapes in abundance. One of these is potassium, the mineral partly responsible for the enthusiasm about grapes among heart specialists. Potassium in balance with sodium is responsible for the necessary electric current running through the body, assuring good energy and a well-functioning brain and nervous system. Potassium for the body is necessary for a strong, trouble-free heart and well-functioning intestines. The wine made from grapes is cautiously suggested, even promoted, for some health problems or as a preventive medicine. The apostle Paul advised the youthful Timothy whom he lovingly called his son: *"... A little wine for thy stomach's sake and thine often infirmities"* (I Timothy 5:23.) Timothy was a sensitive, impassioned, emotional young man. It's understandable that his devoted "father Paul" suggested a common remedy to help him calm down and relax.

Some believers maintain that "wine" means juice of the grape or *fresh* juice. However, realistically considering Bible times when there was no refrigeration, one must recognize that the juice of the harvest soon fermented and was made into wine, nature's way of extending its shelf life. And we know from several Bible accounts that wine, not fresh juice, "lifted the spirits and made men merry." Many people who have lived with a delicate stomach know that "a little wine," as Paul said, a few minutes before eating, can prevent indigestion. Notice Paul said a *little* wine. We truly need to be moderate in all things. *"Let your moderation be known unto all men"* (Philippians 4:5).

Recently physicians and health practitioners have agreed that a daily glass of red wine is good for the heart. The French, who have a high-fat diet and regularly drink red wine, have far fewer heart attacks than Americans. In the making of this wine, the whole grape is used, skin, meat, and seeds. The natural phytochemicals therein work synergistically with other nutrients in the body to further health and performance.

77

Many Bible followers are so troubled by the alcohol in wine that they do not accept drinking it. They cite the admonition by the Apostle Peter "to take no strong drink." Some believers hold that wine is not a strong drink. They classify as strong drink the hard liquors with their greater alcohol content. They drink wine in moderation as the ancient Hebrews and Jesus did.

Taking all of this into consideration, industry is beginning to make wine without alcohol. My question is, How much better will this new product be? Does it contain preservatives? Does it contain the chemical residues used in processing?

In the meantime, there are those among the faithful who drink their mealtime portion of wine. Others are considering taking it or are starting to take it for their hearts since learning about red wine as an aid to avoiding heart disease.

And there are those who ask the question, "How can the wine of today compare with the natural, healthful product of Bible times?" Sulfites and other toxic preservatives and chemicals are used in the processing, all known to be very bad for us. A number of people get headaches from drinking even a small glass of wine.

Many years ago the state of Washington passed a law prohibiting the use of preservatives in the production of wine. This law was little known at the time, because Washington produced only a small amount of wine. A friend of my father's had planted a large vineyard on an island in Washington State with Island Bell grapes, which were developed for the cool, wet climate of Puget Sound. In his newly built winery, the man produced wine uncontaminated by toxic disinfectants, bactericides or preservatives. By assiduous attention to cleanliness, sterilization of vessels and utensils with steam, and pasteurization of the wine, he manufactured a product without the use of toxic substances. As the wine industry grew, however, the government was persuaded to rescind the law in order that Washington wine makers could better compete with neighboring states.

In the last few years some companies have begun making wine again without preservatives. My father would have been pleased. A faithful believer, he attributed the twelve good years added to his already long life to his friend's insistence that he drink a little wine every day. He survived a near fatal heart attack. The wine, a loving gift, was of course from his friend's naturally produced vintages.

In Europe, some Mediterranean countries and South America, it is not uncommon for a physician to prescribe "a little good wine" as a stimulant for an older person. A glass of wine for generations has been prescribed before a meal to a patient with poor digestion. It relaxes the stomach and enhances the digestive process. Wine is also prescribed for some stomach parasites. A few generations ago it was prescribed for tuberculosis. In our nation, where the philosophy prevails that "If a little is good, more is better," many people fear the very real danger of becoming addicted to alcohol from drinking even a little bit every day.

The drinking of wine is perhaps a matter for the individual believer to decide about in his or her own conscience. It is well to keep in mind the Apostle Paul's reminder: *"Don't eat meat or drink wine or do anything else if it might cause a Christian to stumble"* (Romans 14:21, NLT).

How wonderful it is in this over-indulged, technological, unsatisfied "I want more" age that there are many people pursuing the rediscovery of the ancient foods that the earth offers for our sustenance. Several of these have been reintroduced to commerce. In the 1970s and 1980s several dedicated health-conscious people cultivated the seeds of a few pounds of amaranth, an ancient, highly nutritious tasty grain from Mexico, to pre-production levels for the general health food market. *Prevention Magazine* sponsored this project. In a few short years the grain came into production. Now health food stores and co-ops and some supermarkets across the land carry the grain. Other grains from ancient civilizations, some mentioned in the Bible, are also on the market, including teff, spelt and kamut. The latter is the highest in protein of all cereal grains.

Not only grains but also native vegetables figure in the worldwide search: seeds of original potatoes from Peru, native corns of our own Southwestern United States and Mexico and northern parts of South America (Venezuela, Ecuador, Colombia and Peru). Tomatoes and peppers from the Andes have been gathered, planted and put into production. Food analysts have found that they contain much more nutritional value than propagated and domesticated varieties. It is interesting to note that cultivated spinach, even organically grown, has only one-third as much potassium and vitamin A precursor as wild spinach, generally known as lambsquarter, which is a delicious spinach-like green leaf plant growing all over the United States and Mexico, mainly at the edge of cultivated fields.

Of interest also are bell peppers. The original red bell pepper is sweeter, milder in taste, and has far more vitamins—especially vitamin C—carotene and most other nutrients common to it than green bell peppers. The green bells were propagated to stay green and not to ripen, and so in essence are an unnatural variety. Eating green bell peppers is comparable to eating immature green apples. Green bell peppers, like green apples, give a great many people indigestion. Most of our fresh market and superstore produce has been genetically hybridized to yield the largest, best-keeping, most pest-resistant, sweetest-tasting vegetables and fruits for the budget-conscious consumer. The lowering of nutrition through propagation is also true of many varieties of fruits, nuts and seeds that we eat today. It has been found that these propagated varieties cause allergic reactions for many people who have no problem with the original variety. The yellow and orange varieties of the bell pepper fall somewhere in between the ancient red bells, to which few are allergic, and the propagated green one, which many people cannot eat.

When we tamper with the natural order God intended for us, we can experience unpleasantness in all sorts of ways. *"Ye shall keep my statutes. Thou shalt not let thy cattle gender with a diverse kind; thou shalt not sow thy field with mingled seed: neither shall a garment mingled of linen and woolen come upon thee"* (Leviticus 19:19). In other words, God does not like us to tamper with the "seed." That includes both the seed of animals and the seed of plants and fabric sources. One wonders where all of today's research and activity in genetics will lead us. Is it in accordance with God's will?

Under the new covenant, these actions on our part are not sins. However, the quality of the product is often diminished, and we become the loser. We do not reap the full benefit of it. God lets us know that "things" are not intrinsically sinful. It is what we do with them that is sinful. We are allowed to eat the propagated fruits, vegetables, seeds and grains. The problem is that our bodies suffer from being denied the unadulterated completeness of the original food. God has known this all along and has warned us throughout the Scriptures. By not following Him in all things, we short-change ourselves in so many ways.

Chapter Eleven

THE FORGOTTEN SIN

The Scriptures have a special name for overindulgence in foods. It's a name that instantly brings to mind an impression we do not like, an unpleasant image we erase from our inner vision the minute we hear it. Rarely is the word spoken, so distasteful is it. The word is even painful to write. This word is gluttony. Because of its offensiveness to us, we ignore it, the cause for it, and what it stands for. And we fail to recognize the awesomely serious consequences of it. Yet by ignoring gluttony we fall victim to it and suffer the consequences.

The time has come to face the word, to brave an examination of the full meaning, to admit we have brushed it aside. By denying it we have actually become ignorant of its existence and, by default, guilty of committing the very sin of gluttony. It is not difficult to admit that we occasionally, frequently, or usually overeat. There are lots of sympathizers out there, so much so that the act of overeating is often accepted as a normal, expected part of our everyday lives.

Is overeating *really* so bad? Is it truly harmful enough to be classified as a sin? First, let's look at what has been known and, in recent times, discussed.

Many doctors say overeating is the single greatest cause of degenerative disease. It so overloads the capacity of most systems in the body that the various functions these systems perform are either slowed, clogged or even stopped for a time. They become so inefficient in their tasks that whatever digestion and assimilation is done is poor and incomplete. Overeating also contributes to lowering of the immune system.

There's a powerful, well-engineered, quiet-running food-processor on the market that is a joy to operate because of all the things it can do well. However, if it is overloaded and forced to take in even a little bit more than the directions recommend, it can soon be clogged and even lock up in its operation, stopping all production until relieved of its overstuffing. If such careless, irresponsible treatment is continued, the machine breaks down in one or more areas and we have dysfunction.

The body, a complex biological machine, is similar. It is so "fearfully and wondrously made" that it will take a great deal of abuse, oftentimes years and years of it before it noticeably begins to break down. And, quite innocently, when many of us become the victims of this breakdown into disease and crisis we ask, "Why me?" Yet others who abuse their bodies, sometimes worse than we do, continue to appear in good health, functioning normally. However, they too eventually and inevitably suffer insidious body breakdown when they continue their unwise lifestyles. Here are some guidelines sprinkled throughout the Bible to keep us reminded and instructed in how to conduct ourselves:

The answers lie couched in God's word in quiet phrases throughout the Bible.

- Respect the Temple of the Soul, our one and only body. Take care of it. *"Your body is the temple of the Holy Ghost"* (I Corinthians 6:19). Feed it the way God commanded, exercise it with walking or some other form of not-too-strenuous exercise, and give it ample rest by getting seven to eight hours' sleep nightly.
- Be moderate in all things. *"Let your moderation be known unto all men"* (Phillipians 4:5).
- Eat natural, living foods the way God commanded and instructed.
- Eat whole fruits and vegetables, not juices, except for temporary treatment of an illness, to cleanse the body, to end a fast, or to give the body the pleasant treat of a rest from eating.
- Many problems have surfaced since we have become a nation of too much juice drinking.
  A. Juices are incomplete foods. They lack the necessaty, essential fiber of whole fruits and vegetables. As a result, digestion suffers.
  B. Small children who are given two or more glasses of juice a day do not grow normally. They are smaller than average. Their digestive systems do not properly develop. Their strength is below normal. They become more allergy prone. The list goes on and on.
  C. Adults who drink a lot of juice each day at the expense of more complete foods, soon experience lowered health, stamina and energy, plus

weight gain if the juices are made up of mostly fruits. (Juices that contain much fruit sugar contain many calories.)

- Eat very little animal fat. Eat only the meat if you choose animal products. This does not include butter, which is not of the flesh of the animal. *"It shall be a perpetual statute for your generations through out all your dwellings, that ye eat neither fat [flesh fat] nor blood"* (Leviticus 3:17).
- Do not eat the blood (bloodwurst, blood sausage, blood pudding, etc.). *"Ye shall not eat any thing with the blood..."* (Leviticus 19:26).
- "Bitter herbs" grown naturally are used medicinally throughout the Bible. For instance, hyssop was much used because it is good for just about everything, internally and externally: it is a cleanser of the blood, the digestive system, the liver and the lungs; it is a help against mucous, parasites, skin rashes and sore throats; it can be used as a gargle, mouth wash, tea and tonic; and it is a regulator of blood pressure, both high and low. The mold that produces Penicillin grows on hyssop leaves. Bitter herbs have one thing in common, a white crystalline substance that is bitter and converts to vitamin-conserving H_2O_2 when activated by water. *"Purge me with hyssop, and I shall be clean"* (Psalm 51:7). (Remember: H_2O_2—hydrogen peroxide—is cleansing and disinfecting.)
- Vinegar was a common food condiment and a main item in the pharmacopoeia of Old Testament times and ever since. Boaz invited Ruth to share a meal with him: *"... And eat of the bread, and dip thy morsel in the vinegar"* (Ruth 2:14). (Bread dipped

in wine vinegar with a few grains of salt is tasty.) When Jesus was on the cross, someone gave him a vessel of vinegar to minister to him in his terribly wounded state. *". . . And they filled a spunge with vinegar, and put it upon hyssop, and put it to his mouth. When Jesus therefore had received the vinegar, he said, It is finished: and he bowed his head, and gave up the ghost"* (John 19:29–30).

Over-processed food was advised against by the prophet Isaiah when he wrote, "Bread grain is easily crushed, so the farmer doesn't keep on pounding it" (paraphrase of Isaiah 28:28). Bread grains are not very hard. Today's prepared cereal manufacturers "keep on pounding" the cereal grains, pounding and crushing and pressing and breaking down with chemicals, heat and additives of various kinds. Even a form of propyl alcohol may be used to make the product so highly refined, so easy to chew, so taste-lessened that the manufacturers can use artificial and other flavors to give the cereal a sweet, delicate, satisfying flavor that has universal appeal. In all this processing, most nutrients are destroyed and so contaminated with solvents like propyl alcohol (isopropyl, propanol, etc.) that they are not only nutritionally robbed but also cause damage to the liver.

The further we get from God's original products, the fewer are the nutrients and the more likely we are to overeat them. Since we *must* take nourishment to live, God provided the law of supply for the demands of our body, along with this admonition: "Moderation in all things." By not obeying that law and by eating more than the body needs, we overload the system and cause harm to it. If a river receives too much water, the banks and surrounding area are damaged and are never quite the same again. Our bodies are affected in the same way. If they receive too much food and unnatural drink, they are never quite the same. "Too much" destroys them. Remember, many physicians say the single greatest cause of breakdown and destruction in the body is *overeating*.

The Bible calls it gluttony, which God equates with drunkenness. Both gluttony and drunkenness are sins because they are harmful to us. They both displease God and go against His instruction. *". . . This our son is stubborn and rebellious, he will not obey our voice; he is a glutton, and a drunkard. And all men of his city shall stone him with stones, that he die: so shalt thou put evil away from among you . . ."* (Deuteronomy 21:20–21)

Solomon, in the great wisdom of his proverbs, wrote, *"For the glutton and the drunkard shall come to poverty..."* (Proverbs 23:21). Poverty in health, certainly; poverty in financial resources, probably. To our precious bodies, gluttony and drunkenness both do harm and are considered a transgression, an abomination. In other words, a sin. *"Now this was the sin of your sister Sodom: She and her daughters were arrogant, overfed and unconcerned; they did not help the poor and needy. They were haughty and did detestable things before me. Therefore I did away with them as you have seen"* (Ezekiel 16:49–50, NIV). They defied God, were overindulged (gluttonous), indifferent and callous about the care of their bodies, God's temple, besides doing *detestable* things.

If you knew you would get only one automobile in your entire lifetime, how do you suppose you would treat it? I'm sure every consideration would be given it: the best gas, oil, the purest radiator water and a carport or garage to protect it from sun, rain and snow. No jackrabbit starts, but a careful warm-up of the motor on a cold day. You would weigh every aspect of a long trip to avoid undue wear and tear on it, opting in the end to go by bus, plane, boat or train. And the care and consideration you would give the upholstery, the carpets, the paint job, the tires! Everything that could be done to preserve it and keep it at the peak of performance would be done to make it last all through your lifetime.

But what about our body? We feed it anything and everything from the supermarket or deli or the junk food cafe. Without hesitation we eat all things served at restaurants. We celebrate with sweets and alcoholic beverages. Our picnics are highlighted with fat-filled and false foods. For a time we say, "I feel great! My body was made to heal. Of course things happen now and then to some people, but they won't happen to me." Cannot we all identify now and then with these phrases?

Are we reading or ignoring God's word? Don't bad things eventually happen from time to time to all of us? *". . . For he maketh his sun to rise on the evil and on the good, and sendeth rain on the just and on the unjust"* (Matthew 5:45).

It is true, we do a lot for the good of our bodies. We provide the best we can for them—clothing, medical checkups, rest and activity. We see that we get adequate nourishment for normal body functioning and for sustaining what we feel is normal life.

But what about the quality of that life? Oh, we provide the best possible housing (we think. But we may fail to consider the toxic chemicals in the materials we will have to live with for years). Our clothing is the best and we wear special shoes. We have sports and exercise equipment, we take vacations, have diversion times and social intercourse for fun and balance, all carefully and as wisely selected as we know how.

What about what we put into that well-clothed, sheltered, exercised, vacationed body? For foods we make regular trips to the well-stocked supermarkets to satisfy our appetites with those marvelous, prepared, processed, canned, frozen, packaged and preserved foods we buy in *advisable* variety and because they taste so good. They are all beautifully attractive—eye appeal is good for the appetite and for digestion—and they take little or no time to prepare. How we enjoy the supermarkets! We are even truly thankful for them. In His love and mercy our God is the great Provider; He allows us to eat everything they have to offer. No sin there. So there is really no sin to eating, no problem. Our distresses come from other phases and areas of our life. Right? Well . . .

Have we opened Pandora's food box and dumped out the contents? Can we refute the accusation that our highly processed, chemically treated foods have turned us statistically into the sickest of the developed nations?

Morticians tell us that the average elderly corpse is so full of chemicals and drugs that the body can hardly decompose. Some hardly need embalming fluids. Each year those corpses are a little younger than the ones the year before.

No single factor is responsible for bringing this present state of affairs about. Not only have we abused our bodies and neglected the care of them, but we have damaged the very world we live in. We have taken lightly, and many times knowingly ignored, the laws of nature. We are reaping a bitter harvest because of our performance. *". . . Whatsoever a man soweth, that shall he also reap"* (Galatians 6:7). As a beloved pastor recently wrote, "We must all repent and ask for forgiveness. Then we can know peace and joy."

Chapter Twelve

GREAT NUTRITION LESSONS THE SCRIPTURES TEACH

The most exciting truths in the Bible about nutrition are found in the stories of Moses leading the children of Israel out of Egypt, and Daniel as a captive of Babylonian King Nebuchadnezzar.

All of us love to read how God miraculously provided a special food for His people after He led them out of Egypt and through the desert. This food, small, round, and slightly sweet, appeared as the morning fog lifted. Manna was what it was called. It was such a complete, satisfying, tasty food that the body needed nothing else for perfect health and maximum energy. However, after a while the people complained about it. Some even wished they were back in bondage in Egypt where they could have such things as fish, meat, leeks, garlic and spices. This angered a generous, loving God. However, in His permissive will He sent them quail, blown in from the sea in droves, until the birds covered the ground. Everyone gathered at least "ten homers" (about sixty bushels, according to a footnote to Numbers 11:32). What they didn't eat they spread on the ground to dry. But before the meat could be digested, those who had craved this other food and bitterly complained about the manna died.

One can well imagine that in their craving they ate so much that they made themselves deathly sick. This is what can happen when people become overwrought and upset, then gorge on heavy foods, especially when their systems are accustomed to and cleansed by a light, vegetarian diet. They can get acute indigestion and die, either quickly, depending on individual differences, or over a period of time, if they continue to overeat. After that disastrous episode, the Israelites ate manna for the rest of their wandering in the wilderness.

As long as the children of Israel ate the manna God provided, they were without sickness. Their sandals and clothing did not wear out and lasted for all of the forty years of their sojourn in the desert. We've learned that a wrong— not God-recommended—diet, especially in a hot climate, can cause much toxic waste to build up in the body. Those toxins are largely thrown off through the skin by heavy sweating. This toxic sweat soon literally eats through clothing and even leather footwear. By contrast, a clean lifestyle and a pure diet, as manna certainly was, produced no toxin in the sweat to wear out clothing. And since nothing is impossible for God, He was able to extend all their wearing apparel for the full generation. *"And I have led you forty years in the wilderness: your clothes are not waxen old upon you, and thy shoe is not waxen old upon thy foot"* (Deuteronomy 29:5–6).

The story of Daniel teaches an even more understandable, practical lesson in food. When King Nebuchadnezzar ordered Daniel and his three companions, Shadrach, Meshach and Abednego, to eat at his table, Daniel balked. He declared in his heart that he would not defile himself with the "portion of the king's meat," nor with his wine. Ashpenaz, the master of the king's eunuchs, who was pleased with the appearance and character of the four young Israeli princes, replied to Daniel that he would be in danger of losing his head for not obeying the king's command. But Daniel persisted, saying to Melzar, whom the prince of eunuchs had set over the four, *"Prove thy servants, I beseech thee, ten days; and let them give us pulse to eat, and water to drink"* (Daniel 1:12).

Melzar agreed. *". . . At the end of the ten days their countenances appeared fairer and fatter in flesh than all the children [youths of the court] which did eat the portion of the king's meat. Thus Melzar took away the portion of their meat, and the wine that they should drink; and gave them pulse"* (Daniel 1:15–16).

And what was pulse? Various Bible dictionaries define it as grains, seeds and legumes. But the word pulse really means beat, throb, flow of life. We can feel the flow of blood in the wrist when we want to count the heartbeat. In grains and seeds, pulse is the germination, which means the flow of life that has come into the seed. It is the early sprout or bud after water has activated life in the dormant grain. Soaked in fresh water overnight, the dormant grains and seeds come to life as they absorb the moisture. Drained, washed, drained again and set aside in a draining position, that life in the grains starts growing. After about forty-eight hours of this process two or three times a day, the tiny growth is the length of the seed itself and the living grains are ready to eat.

Their nutrition has increased from eight to two hundred times. They can be eaten raw when warmed in a double boiler and served as cooked rice with a sprinkle of pure sea salt. They are delicious and satisfying as whole grain cereal or blended as a porridge, or they can be ground in a food grinder, formed into flat loaves, and "baked" in the sun for one to three hours, as was the custom extant in the Middle East before and during Daniel's time. This sun baking starts the process of fermentation, nature's oldest form of extending shelf life. A product reportedly developed by the ancient Sumarians, it was eaten by Daniel and his companions.

Sprouted seeds and grains can be a complete diet, maintaining health, energy, and a long disease-free life. Legumes were first sprouted, then used in several ways. Lentil sprouts are quite tasty in the crisp raw form, served alone or with other vegetables. Others of the bean-pea family are tastier cooked. Another reason for sprouting is that all dry seeds, grains and legumes, which become fresh *vegetables* when sprouted, take very little time to cook (five to ten minutes). That was a significant saving of fuel in the Holy Land where wood was so scarce people cooked and baked using mostly animal dung for fuel.

The apostles walked everywhere with Jesus and in their continuing ministries after His crucifixion and ascension into Heaven. Often their meals were made up of grains in the immature state, which they picked as they walked through fields. Nothing could have been better for them. Those before-harvest–time seeds provided complete nutrition and were full of all the natural vitamins. They were rich in minerals, protein and digestible (raw) starch, replete with enzymes, and contained cleansing, sustaining, energy-giving oxygen. Those tough and tasty grains needed a lot of chewing. The act of mastication not only stimulated the brain, but it also generated plenty of digestive juices in the mouth that, when thoroughly mixed with food and swallowed, stimulated the production of stomach acid (hydrochloric acid) to assure good digestion of the protein and to kill parasites in the stomach before they reached the intestines where they caused diarrhea. This food provided complete nutrition and was totally satisfying to the appetite. By requiring a lot of chewing, it discouraged overeating.

Although the diet of Bible times may appear to be meager, especially in variety, it actually had all the basics of our diet today. People then didn't take every product, large or small, and extend it into complicated recipes. Today, through alterations, innovations and mixtures with other foods, industry has reached the point where it is obsessed with selling more to people than is good for them.

We have gone far afield of the wholesome, delightful, satisfying simplicity of natural foods. A look at some of the foods eaten by mankind in Bible times can perhaps give a few surprises. Many grains were grown in Israel and in surrounding countries, including wheat, spelt, millet, barley, oats, teff and kamut. Ground into flours, they were sometimes sifted to remove some of the covering of the seed to make a fine, nearly white flour for such special occasions as feast days, birthdays, weddings and anniversaries. Bread, with or without oil and leavening, could be made into loaves, rolls, thin cakes or small dried crackers. Cakes sweetened with honey or crude sugar were made for festivities, feasts and special celebrations. They were treats, *not daily fare.*

Historians wrote about the crystallized juice of cane (crude sugar) as early as the days of Alexander the Great (356–323 B.C.). A brilliant, imaginative, practical thinker and idea man, Alexander, according to Greek historians, sneaked sugar into the vast ranks of the enemy after dark one night. The soldiers, gorging on such a rare bonanza, became so stimulated with energy that they hardly slept. Alexander and his troops moved in before dawn. They had little difficulty fighting an army weakened with the after effects of gorging on a sweet ordinarily used as a condiment. It made them, in a few hours, so lethargic that they had neither the will nor the stamina nor the strength to fight. Alexander easily won the battle.

The ancient Hebrews also made raisin cakes and fig bars, as well as combinations of fruits for confections and treats for notable occasions or gifts.

Many fruits are mentioned in the Scriptures—apples, grapes, raisins, figs, pomegranates and dates. Numerous historians and Bible scholars believe that royalty and the rich may have had pitted fruits like peaches, cherries, plums, and apricots on occasion. These fruits were mentioned in Greek, Roman, Persian, Egyptian and Chinese writings that date back to centuries before Christ. Pears, of which there is a record claiming to date back to at least six thousand years ago, grew in a variety of climates. Today Israel produces several kinds of luscious pears.

Herbs grew in great variety. They included a broad spectrum of plants and trees that provided edible leaves, stems, roots, seeds, and pods. One such plant is carob, the pod of the locust tree, the food John the Baptist ate in the wilderness along with wild honey. Herbs provided spices, condiments and substances, all of which helped to make up a supply of nutrients that spanned the four seasons of the year. It is said that the diet of people in the Scriptures included two hundred different items. Throughout the course of a year, the number of foods they ate far exceeded the number of foods in the average American's conventional diet of forty to fifty. Studies today of the average teenager's diet of junk foods show that he or she eats less than twenty different food items, greatly below the vast number of foods God created and provided for us to eat.

Then of course there was the flesh of many herbivorous animals, fish and fowl. The masses in villages, towns and cities ate little flesh because of quick spoilage and high cost. Eggs and milk of goats and cattle rounded out the long list of edibles allowed by God for all of His people.

It is interesting to observe, as I have pointed out, that God's original instruction on what to eat—fruits with their seeds as told in Genesis 1:29—is in the first chapter of the first book of the Bible. And His last awesome words on what our food will be during the millennium on the reconstituted earth, where Jesus Messiah will reign as King of kings and Lord of lords, appear in the last chapter of the last book of the Bible: *". . . and on either side of the river, was there the tree of life, which bare twelve manner of fruits, and yielded her fruit every month: and the leaves of the tree were for the healing of the nations"* (Revelation 22:2).

There is nothing in God's way of eating to cause a weight problem, whether over or underweight. When we do not eat this way and become overweight or underweight, we are under bondage to *weight* and under the *weight* of bondage. And we get sick. God is the only One Who can free us and heal us completely.

Chapter Thirteen

DOES OUR CHOICE
OF FOODS LEAD US ASTRAY?

Solomon, the wisest of men, wrote much about the wisdom of what, when and how much to eat. In Deuteronomy Moses gave meaningful instruction, and Paul left reminders in a couple of remarkable statements that apply to healthy eating. Most of these have already been quoted.

Learning what and how to eat is actually, for most of us, *un*learning, *re*learning and *practice* learning.

It goes without saying that we accept the fact that we have to eat. It is God's will that we eat. We give thanks that we can eat and have something to eat. So we really eat to glorify God. Eating sustains and takes care of the body, the temple of the soul and spirit. "*. . . He that eateth, eateth to the Lord, for he giveth God thanks*" (Romans 14:6).

If we eat to glorify God, then we recognize, thank and praise Him *first.* That's why we say grace, our heartfelt gratitude to a Father Who provides for His children. Before the time of Christ, the Jewish people said grace *after* the meal. *"The Lord is my shepherd; I shall not want"* (Psalm 23:1). It is an affirmation, a giving of thanks after the fact. It is appreciation. Again God assures us that His people who follow Him do not go hungry. Not only are we not to abuse our bodies with wrong food or with too much, but we are also not to abuse our food—overheat, overprocess or overkill it. God covets our appreciation of food, our respect for it, our enjoyment of it, our not wasting what He has laid before us. Therefore, we are truly to eat to please Him. That is the main issue. In the grace we offer we need to review the matter, pray in the Spirit, pray God's word over the food, and ask Him to bless it to its intended use of health, strength, and energy. Then we can eat it...

- to please Him
- to nourish our bodies
- to enjoy the gift of food.

He not only blesses the food, He blesses us too. And we are to bless Him. God is pleased when we bless Him. David blessed Him often, as in Psalm 103:1: *"Bless the Lord, O my soul: and all that is within me, bless his holy name."*

How sad it is that we too often abuse the privilege of being in God's grace and having our food needs met, by (1) overeating or gorging, or (2) wolfing down those precious foods without appreciation. This is why we should not eat if we are anxious or in a rush or depressed to the point of failing to respect the God-given privilege of eating. Such emotions cause us to eat without properly chewing, which leads to stomach disorders and poor digestion and elimination. Eating rapidly causes some people to overeat, which, as we know, is gluttony, and gluttony is wrong-doing.

You may be thinking, "Avoid eating a meal because I'm a bit upset, or in a hurry or pressured? It's not good to skip meals. I'll get a headache or become weak. I'll suffer deficiencies." But didn't God assure us of His constant care if we trust and follow Him? *"The Lord will not suffer the soul of the righteous to famish . . ."* (Proverbs 10:3).

Not infrequently the pressure of my schedule makes it advisable for me to skip a meal. For the most part, I never miss it. Sometimes it's dinner I have to skip because of an early evening lecture. I do not eat afterwards before going to bed. A late meal may mean poor sleep and disturbing dreams. Eating nothing allows the body and the mind to rest and get up refreshed, with energy and a joyous anticipation of the breakfast of fruit God so graciously provided.

If a person is physically unable to skip a meal, he needs to concentrate on health and pray for guidance in learning how better to care for it. Having a reaction due to not eating the next meal or a between-meal snack means he probably suffers from hypoglycemia (low blood sugar). When we learn what foods give any sort of unpleasant reaction, we must completely avoid eating them. Leaving off all such foods will in time allow the body to heal, to go without food comfortably for a meal or two, and eventually to be able to tolerate the once-offending food. So let us seek the knowledge of our food sensitivities and allergies and the wisdom to deal with them. When Solomon asked God for wisdom and knowledge and not *"riches, wealth, or honor, nor the life of thine enemies, neither . . . long life,"* (II Chronicles 1:11), God granted them all. He will do the same for us.

We need to eat to satisfy ourselves, not stuff ourselves. *"The good man [or woman or child] eats to live, while the evil man lives to eat"* (Proverbs 13:25, LB) *"The backslider gets bored with himself; the Godly man's life is exciting"* (Proverbs 14:14, LB). When we dedicate our eating to God, there's a whole new emphasis on it and on Him. We please Him when we recognize His wishes and take care of His temple. We are not eating primarily to please ourselves. But by eating the quality and quantity that please Him, we enjoy the by-product of pleasing ourselves. We are satisfied. And with that satisfaction there is contentment, peace and a good digestion.

An essential first act in the feeding and care of our body is to *take the bad out of the diet.* This cannot be overemphasized. The bad means junk food, processed, overcooked, artificially flavored and additive foods. They are exactly the opposite of the *natural* foods God ordered—natural fruits, vegetables, seeds, nuts and grains. And if one is not a vegetarian, then eat moderate amounts of naturally raised animal products in addition.

Ask the Lord for a vision of an active, well-proportioned you, one who feels and looks spirited and bright. Then when you begin a meal, bring that vision to mind. Let your food suggest that vision, and if you are alone keep it before you as you eat. If you're eating with others present, talk about uplifting things, pleasant happenings, an enjoyable incident, a restful vacation. Or discuss the Scriptures as they apply to your everyday life, your hopes, plans, dreams. Or report some little triumph of the day, or carry on light-hearted, pleasant chat in fun and merriment.

Avoid all discussions of trials, failures, frustrations or disappointments. They are past. Dead. Gone. We are to leave them there, buried and forgotten. Live this moment anticipating the next, knowing God is with you. If you persist in dredging up the past, except as a point of reference only, God will stand back, letting you dredge alone.

But keep Him by your side, in your heart, on your mind. Then enjoy! Be thankful for the moment. If alone, enjoy that aloneness in peace and quiet and fellowship with God and the Holy Spirit. Talk out loud to Them. Be thankful for fellowship if you're with others. Is there tension? Dissension? Remain quiet. Breathe deeply and eat slowly. Smile. Jesus said, "Be calm and know that I am God."

If food doesn't taste good, stop eating it. Don't continue for the sake of appearances or habit. Try to look pleasant. Pray under your breath. In case of verbal conflict around you, repeat the name of Jesus. Say it over and over to yourself.

Watch your intake of sweets, white flour foods, hydrogenated cooking fats, and flesh meats. Bible translators have frequently translated the Greek and Hebrew words for *victuals, substance, food, nourishment* and *rations* as meat, which to those of us speaking English usually means flesh meat. Because of this, many readers of English language versions are led to believe that people throughout the Scriptures ate far more meat than they actually did. You will recall that only immediately after the Flood was a great amount of meat eaten. That was because there remained for a time after the Flood little else, if anything at all, to eat.

It is probable that Noah and his family found some edible roots, but surely only enough to supplement their diet of flesh.

That interval, the only time of heavy meat eating recorded in the Bible, was an emergency, not an example of a diet to follow.

Remember Solomon's words: *"Do not join those who drink too much wine or gorge themselves on meat"* (Proverbs 23:20, NIV). (This time the ancient Hebrew word for meat means flesh meat.)

Sugar is also addictive. It is the most addictive of all edibles, partly because mankind has a natural affinity to sweet things, an inborn taste for sweets. Proverbs alerts us: *"It is not good to eat much honey . . ."* (Proverbs 25:27).

Again, the Bible warns us about sweets. They are called delicacies, which today means pastries, pies, cakes, cookies, candies, etc. *"When thou sittest to eat with a ruler [official, person of recognized authority], consider diligently what is before thee: And put a knife to thy throat, if thou be a man given to appetite [gluttony]. Be not desirous of his dainties: for they are deceitful meat"* (Proverbs 23:1–3). (Meat here meant victuals in the original Hebrew text.)

Why does God warn us so many times about eating meat when He allows it? Remember, He is a gracious God, and no "thing" He created is intrinsically bad. The bad comes from what we do with it. That is God's great concern. That is why He makes such strong statements all through Solomon's writings, such as, "Put a knife to thy throat." Gluttony is that serious.

God recommends that we eat all or mostly vegetarian fare. That's the perfect fuel He originally planned and provided for the body. The organs of digestion were not designed to accept another type of fuel. The combustion engine of a car was designed to run on gasoline but can run inefficiently on kerosene. The body, designed to run on plants, can run on animal matter; however, it runs inefficiently and for a shorter time. As the car motor would eventually clog with unburned substances from the kerosene, so the body eventually becomes clogged with undigested substances from flesh meat.

So we begin to understand why and how the Scriptures teach us the correct way to eat for total health, prevention, longevity and energy.

Nothing we do for our physical being is more important than nutrition. That's why God focused His first commandment on food in the first chapter of the first book of the Bible. Because they disobeyed God in the area of eating, Adam and Eve were turned out of their beautiful homeland.

Undisciplined eating got Esau into trouble. His out-of-control appetite and demand for a bowl of lentil stew caused him to lose his birthright.

The prophet Eli so overindulged his love of food that he became obese, a condition that eventually caused his death. So much weight on his aging body made him awkward and he fell off a stool, an accident so serious for an obese person that it caused a fatal injury. Not only was he uncontrolled in his eating, but he also did not control his two sons who became as fat as he.

Belshazzar caused his own death prematurely as a result of riotous eating and drinking.

Overeating is a deep-seated habit that keeps many people enslaved. Faint not! The Scriptures also teach us how to break the habit. Read on!

Chapter Fourteen

What Specific Words Teach Biblical Nutrition?

Faced with the need to change our eating habits to fol low Scriptural teaching for quality survival, we need to pray in the Spirit. But how do we do this? An effective start is to read Paul's words: *"Likewise the Spirit also helpeth our infirmities: for we know not what we should pray for as we ought: but the Spirit itself maketh intercession for us with groanings which cannot be uttered"* (Romans 8:26).

The word infirmity means weakness. Isn't it like our Father to provide for every need! For those with eating problems, it is well to pray before a meal. Pray in the Spirit when you go near the refrigerator or pass a cupboard full of snack foods. Repeat the name of Jesus when you are desperately tempted to grab a candy bar. Solomon provided a Scripture that gives the key to eating correctly: *"The righteous eateth to the satisfying of his soul: but the belly of the wicked shall want"* (Proverbs 13:25). And another true bit of wisdom from the wisest man of all times: *"The full soul loatheth an honeycomb; but to the hungry soul every bitter thing is sweet"* (Proverbs 27:7). Note: A modern-day deficiency of the mineral chromium is a major cause of the craving for sweets and the compulsion to overeat. This deficiency may be inexpensively corrected with an over-the-counter mineral supplement.

The soul is made up of mind, personality and emotions. The "full soul" the verse above speaks of refers to supportive, sound emotions and a mind active with worthwhile thoughts and plans. That soul-mind is busily occupied. Such fulfilled, achieving people have little time for thinking about food or compulsive yearning for sweets. How good it is to keep both mind and body busy—busy with work, prayer, reading, spending time with friends and family, helping someone, spending time with a shut-in, having thoughts of doing and accomplishing, doing gardening and hard work.

There is an often-overlooked reason people eat too much: an underactive body and a mind that doesn't have enough to think about constructively, gainfully. Solomon's wisdom brings this to light: *"Slothfulness casteth into a deep sleep; and an idle soul shall suffer hunger"* (Proverbs 19:15).

In other words, an idle, undisciplined soul finds that everything tastes good. In apathy and the absence of challenging thoughts and activities, he will eat unappetizing, ill-tasting, even bitter foods. And good foods he will tend to wolf down and overeat.

God takes pleasure in a gainfully occupied body and an alert mind full of His Word. Such a state of living is satisfying—a term used frequently throughout Scripture. Satisfaction in things physical, mental, emotional and spiritual is a blessing, a pleasant result of living in His will. It is a necessary part of joy. And the joy of the Lord is our strength. How do we get that joy? By pledging (committing) our lives to obeying Him.

There is another reason for eating correct foods. They will strengthen the right attitude toward eating. This is the *setting apart* of your food. The Bible calls it sanctifying. In your mind, ask God to help you set apart the things He instructed you to eat, the things you have decided to eat, the things that will please Him.

The backup for this is found in I Timothy 4:3-5: *"Forbidding to marry, and commanding to abstain from meats, which God hath created to be received with thanksgiving of them which believe and know the truth. For every creature of God is good, and nothing to be refused, if it be received with thanksgiving:For it is sanctified [set apart] by the word of God and prayer."*

It is clear we do not have to be vegetarians. However, we are warned not to be riotous eaters of flesh: *"Be not among winebibbers; among riotous eaters of flesh: For the drunkard and the glutton shall come to poverty: and drowsiness [from gluttony] shall clothe a man with rags"* (Proverbs 23:20-21).

Since the time Esau's craving for food caused him to sell his birthright, mankind has had to contend with persistent, unruly appetite. It is so powerful that it can easily become compulsive. That is why there are so many warnings, so many bits and pieces of advice and help and information on the consequences of letting appetite rule our lives. *"And put a knife to thy throat, if thou be a man of appetite"* (Proverbs 23:2). Happily, fresh raw vegetables are delightful, refreshing, energizing and satisfying. They do not cause an out-of-control, *binge-tinged* appetite. Putting a knife to the throat is a bit drastic. One person told me she drew an outline on a piece of paper of her sharpest chopping knife. Then she folded it along the cutting side and slid it across her throat when she was tempted to eat a helping of a rich dessert. "It worked," she said. "My sub-conscious got the message and I was able to say no."

We are frequently, unwaveringly encouraged in our walk: *". . . But he that is of a merry heart hath a continual feast"* (Proverbs 15:15).

A Scripture I love to repeat for its focus on a wonderful, helpful, comforting prayer is this: *"Keep falsehood and lies far from me; give me neither poverty nor riches, but give me only my daily bread"* (Proverbs 30:8, NIV). (Bread here means all kinds of substance: food for the body, mind and soul.) This helps to maintain a balance of physical food, spiritual food and food for thought. It has stopped some of us from gorging on fudge cake or ice cream or peanut but-ter cookies.

The book of Deuteronomy contains a few profoundly helpful verses: *"And he will love thee, and bless thee, and multiply thee: he will also bless the fruit of thy womb, and the fruit of thy land, thy corn, and thy wine, and thine oil, the increase of thy kine [cattle], and the flocks of thy sheep, in the land which he sware unto thy fathers to give thee. Thou shalt be blessed above all people: there shall not be male or female barren among you, or among your cattle. And the Lord will take away from thee all sickness, and will put none of the evil diseases of Egypt, which thou knowest, upon thee; but will lay them upon all them that hate thee"* (Deuteronomy 7:13–15, KJV).

Fortunately, we have the *Word* to help us choose right food: food that pleases God. It tastes good, it nourishes us, it satisfies us and keeps our bodies at a correct weight with a wonderful supply of energy. The Old Testament gave us fruits and vegetables, seeds (nuts and grains), sprouts, honey, the milk and butter of cattle and goats and a little flesh meat. Eating these natural, balanced foods in moderation keeps our bodies at their natural weight.

In the words of Paul, the New Testament refers much to grain breads, both leavened and unleavened. Before and during the time of Christ, grain breads made up the bulk of the diet. It is interesting to note that there was a lot of sickness and disability among the Israelites of that period, especially in light of recent nutritional observations and discoveries. For several decades our national health has been fraught with illness, and it still is today. Most of us have something wrong with our health, some disease, some physical problem. Since the turn of the century, we have eaten wheat in great quantities, daily and in a fractionated form (white, bleached flour) largely to the exclusion of vegetables, seeds, fruits, legumes and other grains. We are suffering the consequences of this unbalanced diet. *Allergists report that about 90 percent of the population, as a result, are allergic to wheat and wheat products.* When the germ and the bran are stripped from the grain, only about 15 percent of the nutrition remains. That woefully deficient flour is daily made into soft doughy bread and all sorts of sugar-sweetened cakes, pies, pastries, cookies, exotic desserts and confections. Most of those products contain animal fats or hydrogenated (nutritionless) fats and oils, further causing deficiencies, a major contributing factor to degenerative disease, overweight, and obesity.

There is a correlation between the health of today and that of the Holy Land two thousand years ago. Is it fine, white flour. They made it by grinding wheat very fine and sifting out the bran and germ, the source of vitamin E, minerals and essential fiber. Hebrew people greatly valued this fine white flour for temple sacrifices and for delicacies for their celebrations. One wonders if they gave the "coarse stuff" to the animals, as we did here in America from the turn of the century to the 1920s. My father, a wheat farmer with lots of livestock, supplemented his animals' food with the bran and wheat germ "waste," with good results. What he should also have done was feed some to his scrawny little Elizabeth.

Whole grain breads have healthily sustained people all over the world since time began. The best are sprouted grain breads. They contain all nutrients in abundance. Eaten with the other fresh products God created, mankind can live in health well beyond the seventy to eighty years spoken of in the Scriptures.

Here are the high spots to review to help you change eating habits and regain or maintain the figure you visualize or have and want to keep.

- Rebuke the power of food in your life.
- Eat to please God (and eat His foods).
- Pray before going to the table.
- State what you expect your foods to do for you before you eat: to satisfy your appetite, nourish you, be a blessing to your body, which is God's temple.
- Avoid eating heavy foods when depressed or upset.
- Turn bad eating habits over to the Lord. *"Casting all your care upon Him; for He careth for you"* (I Peter 5:7).
- Discipline your intake of meats (flesh foods) and sweets.

- Remember: You eat to satisfy your needs, *not to stuff yourself.*
- Drink a large glass of water a little while before you eat. (It cleanses and satisfies, and it diminishes your appetite by partially filling your stomach).
- Memorize this Scripture: *"Whether therefore ye eat, or drink, or whatsoever ye do, do all to the glory of God"* (I Corinthians 10:31).

Chapter Fifteen

LEAVES FOR THE HEALING OF THE NATIONS

How beautifully the Scriptures teach us to live and take care of our bodies. It was not intended to be difficult, to take a lot of time and be a heavy burden or even a time-consuming chore. What is taught is a simple way of life. When we follow that prescribed lifestyle, it not only sustains us without undue effort, it is also a joyous experience of freedom from the demanding preparation of complicated, elaborate meals. It helps release us from excessive wants and longings for more and more clothes, expensive furniture, bigger homes, newer cars and so on. Just by following God's way and enjoying His promises, we avoid much anxiety from futile desires for material things. It lessens troubles, frees us from sickness and cuts down on needless extra work and stress. And it saves us money.

Let me hasten to add that choosing His way does not mean we are not going to experience adversity of some kind by way of accident, illness, loss, emotional upheavals, stress, and even death of loved ones. These things come upon all kinds of people, for we are all human and God is no respecter of persons. However, He helps us through all such things if we put Him first in our lives. He sustains us through suffering. He gives us understanding, patience, blessings, hope and assurance. He says, *". . . I will never leave thee, nor forsake thee"* (Hebrews 13:5). Again He assures us: *". . . And, lo, I am with you alway, even unto the end of the world"* (Matthew 28:20).

How does He take care of us? By our asking the Lord to help us, then trusting and praising Him. Obeying Him. Doing our part. By our taking the responsibility for our own health. We select our food from a long list of available natural foods; we eat to nourish the temple of our soul, God's temple. If we defile God's temple by wrong eating and unhealthy living (bad treatment of the body) God will destroy. He does not just say He will destroy our health. Note that He says, *". . . Him shall God destroy"* (I Corinthians 3:16–17).

This is what we are seeing today. People are destroying themselves, and not just their bodies but their minds and spirits as well. They have poor memory, lack of concentration and Alzheimer's disease. Eventually, wrong eating and living destroys the whole person.

In so doing people are killing themselves. It is actually mass suicide.

Drastic? Overstated? Of course not. We see it every day, people dying of degenerative diseases, brought on for the most part by what they put into their bodies.

How do we turn our lives around? What can we do to help the body heal itself? Blessedly, many things. Not only are there healing foods, as has been pointed out, but there is also the natural pharmacopoeia since the beginning of man's walk on and struggle with the earth. And there is help available from physicians who use nutrition, herbalists, and all kinds of able therapists of many disciplines dedicated to natural healing.

To begin, there are the bitter herbs spoken of in Scripture, bitter herbs with the white crystalline element that forms H2O2 (hydrogen peroxide), when water is added. Because of that and other substances, these herbs are exceptionally healing. Optimal oxygen in the body keeps the blood pure and clean. Oxygen is the bottom line in healing and recovery. It's in the blood. If the blood carries plenty of oxygen, the cells do not become diseased. They do not die prematurely. They cannot mutate into cancer cells.

Additional familiar herbs that are naturally bitter and so help oxygenate the blood are dandelion, quinine (extremely bitter and for generations, the only known medicine for treating, alleviating and even curing malaria), chaparral, golden seal and pau d'arco, to name a few. The Bible speaks of bitter herbs, hyssop being the main one. Wild hyssop that grew and still grows today on the dry hillsides and climes of the Promised Land was bitter, though not so much as some other herbs. When cultivated, it is only mildly bitter. Most domesticated plants are milder in taste and less potent than the wild ones. However, they are still effective, especially when used raw (not heated to boiling or pasteurization temperatures).

Carob seed pods of the wild locust tree were not only a pleasant, semi-sweet food, but also a medicine good for the digestion and for the cleansing and normal elimination of wastes from the body. John the Baptist, by living vigorously and healthily on carob, made it famous for all time. Honey, as we mentioned earlier, was promised for Jesus the Messiah by the Old Testament prophet Isaiah. These two foods, in moderation, sharpen the mind to function clearly, optimally. For this reason, they are, in a very real sense, spiritual foods.

Since ancient times, vinegar has been used for health and healing. It is a mild antiseptic. We find it mentioned first in the Old Testament in the book of Numbers. The Lord told Moses how to instruct any person who wanted to separate himself to the Lord through a Nazarite vow. *"He shall separate himself from wine and strong drink, and shall drink no vinegar of wine, or vinegar of strong drink* (for medicinal purposes. When a medicine is used, it does not allow the body to cleanse and purify itself), *neither shall he drink any liquor of grapes, nor eat moist grapes, or dried"* (Numbers 6:3). The length of the vow lasted from eight days to a month. It was a real sacrifice to give up grapes and all the products made from them. Paul and a few others took the vow for a short while. Only Samson and John the Baptist took it for life, the former breaking it and so contributing to his downfall and death.

Another property of vinegar is its mild acidity which protects the body against bacterial and viral disease and helps it recover from disease. Medical science tells us all degenerative diseases occur when the acid/alkaline balance, called the pH, is over on the alkaline side of neutral, which is 7.0. When the body, as nature intended, is slightly on the acid side (between 6.4 and 5.5), bacteria and viruses cannot multiply or proliferate.

By taking two to six or eight teaspoons of vinegar (apple cider vinegar is best for us today) in water a day, we can oftentimes effectively ward off colds and flu. It is also an

118

aid to digestion when stomach acid is low, since it can help the acid in the stomach to digest protein. One other very important fact: the mantle of the skin is normally slightly acid. If it weren't, man would be seriously threatened with infection by every little cut, scratch or burn. Vinegar, used both internally and externally, is an aid to maintaining resistance to disease. Books have been written on vinegar and its effectiveness.

Another thing the ancients knew about and used was silver. A silver coin in a bowl of fresh milk would nearly double the amount of time it could remain fresh. Pioneers and earlier settlers, according to my grandmother, who was one, dropped a shiny silver dollar in a gallon crock of milk and stirred it occasionally to keep it sweet twice as long. People quit using silver coins in milk as ice boxes, then refrigerators, came into use.

The ancient Egyptians, Greeks, Romans, Hebrews and Arabs knew that silver vessels for cooking, eating and drinking helped them avoid sickness and gave them strength. Finger rings of gold (also a beneficial metal) and especially silver were known to protect health. However, only rulers, high officials and rich people who did no physical work could afford to lower their energy by wearing rings on the index finger. The least energy is lost by a metal ring when worn on the third finger. For this reason, the third finger long ago became the universally approved finger for wearing the wedding band. There have been and still are many cultures where the wedding band is worn for life and never taken off. Many ancient peoples also knew that metal completely circling any part of the body lessened the energies, especially those circling the waist (near the naval) and the index finger.

119

How easy it is to let the wisdom of the ages, even as recorded in the Bible, slip into the background and eventually into oblivion. And how exciting it is to resurrect it and find that it is true and still works subtly for our good today.

Chapter Sixteen

WHAT DO THE SCRIPTURES SAY ABOUT FEEDING OUR CHILDREN?

How strange is the land we live in! We worry, we fret, we work hard, we seek answers for the food our children will eat. Then we ask *them* what they want for breakfast. They may not tell us, but they usually do. When they do, we prepare it for them—packaged orange juice, crispy, sugary dry cereal, a glass of homogenized milk, maybe fried strips of bacon. They run off to school or the sandbox or to play their latest CD or cassette. They've had a good, balanced breakfast. Or so it is commonly thought.

But how truly nourishing was it? Was it all natural as God instructed us? Did we follow Him in teaching that to our children? Let's look at each food we let them have.

The juice was far from the original orange: squeezed and partially destroyed by reducing to concentrate, then frozen or killed with heat, then packaged and sealed, the whole process destroying most of the food value. Vitamin C, enzymes and oxygen especially are ruined. The juice, devoid of fiber, pitifully lacked the full nourishment and delightful flavor of the whole, fresh orange. Little was left in the juice except the liquid, fruit sugar and a few precious minerals.

The cereal? On the box are listed the minerals, the vitamins, the protein, the high fiber. Those nutrients are all there in the raw grains before processing. After grinding, mixing with water, forming into flakes or "biscuits" or circles or whatever, treating with chemicals, adding condiments, flavorings and sugar, then toasting in hot ovens, what is left?

To continue, the facts about milk must be exposed. It is homogenized, which means the cream molecule is so changed—made into such fine particles—that the body cannot metabolize it; it is far different from the whole, natural molecules of raw milk. Those broken down, distorted molecules cannot be digested by the body because they are foreign to it and get left in the bloodstream. They end up getting stuck on the blood vessel walls and becoming, according to biochemists, the greatest single cause of heart disease; they are phospholipids that clog the bloodstream. Yes, it can happen even in children.

The strip of bacon is not only indigestible because of the overheated animal fat, but the Bible says we are not to eat it. Pork is called "unclean," because of trichinosis, a parasite that inhabits the tissues of the muscles of the pig. Today, in the curing process with nitrites, sulfites and commercial salt, pork products are all toxic. Poison. Harmful. Difficult to digest and even more difficult to totally eliminate from the body.

We would not think of giving such meals to an animal. Veterinarians say no to bacon for pets. The cereals take no effort to prepare and serve. Consistently given, they could soon cause sickness and death to those innocent creatures.

Even when parents know sugared cereal is not good for their children, they let them have it. The children want it, demand it. How very often we hear mothers say, even in the presence of their children, "My children won't eat this or that; they are very picky. They will eat only certain things." After hearing this, the child, more than ever, demands his own way.

Since when did God say parents should obey their children? How did the authority in the home get shifted from the parents to the children? Many times have you heard mothers say, "My parents made me take a little bit of everything on the table. I had to sit there until I ate it whether I liked it or not. I learned to eat and like just about everything."

Everyone has either seen, known about or experienced the general breakdown of the home since the 1950s. Discipline has broken down. There is failure to communicate, to consider one another, to observe moral standards, to be loyal to each other, to forgive, to do each one's share, to set aside selfish wants for the good of the family. Present in such situations is the refusal to take responsibility, to discipline, to control the self, to try to please each other, and to *not complain*. All these factors are painfully familiar, wearing, and wearying. So it is that we are tempted to not bring up one more thing to an already stressed parent. However, the issue is before us, existing against God's will, becoming worse with each month and year and with increasingly bad effects. An integral part of the problem is junk food and drinks and parents who provide it and permit it.

Here is the present scenario: Children are eating largely junk food. It is advertised on TV, radio and billboards. Children become addicted to it because that's what they have mostly eaten, what their peers eat. They get it at school, at nurseries, at churches, picnics, even at the home of grandparents. They are rewarded by being taken to the fast foods restaurant, a junk food Mecca. Their birthdays are frequently celebrated there. At parties they invariably get cake, ice cream, candy and soft drinks. And all too often they are allowed cookies and other sweets before bed.

Most of these foods are entirely processed. The buns, sandwich breads, pastas, pizzas, cookies, pies and cakes are of chlorine-bleached white flour. The sugar in these products is nothing but empty calories. Sugar shuts down the immune system. The hamburger is made of beef raised unnaturally with antibiotics, steroids and hormones, then slaughtered after being tranquilized and inoculated with chemicals to make it bleed rapidly and to preserve it. Hot dogs usually contain nitrites and sulfites to preserve them. Many times white flour is used as a filler in the wieners. With their spices and condiments they are hard to digest and are not suitable food for the human body, especially for our children.

A concerned third grade teacher of many years' experience and observation volunteered to give examples of two types of behavior she deals with every day. She had talked with the single parent of a hyperactive, attention-deficit pupil who frequently missed school because of colds, stomach flu and ear infection. Here's what she learned: For breakfast the child routinely ate sweet rolls, 7UP or a packaged orange drink, sugar-sweetened dry cereal, white bread toast (he wouldn't eat whole grain bread), and margarine and jelly. Note: Sugar and the artificial flavor and color in the orange drink and the margarine are known to cause hyperactivity in children, and contribute, along with white flour, to decreasing the attention span.

The other example given by the concerned teacher was of an eight-year-old girl whose mother had come to open house for parents. The child rarely missed school for sickness. She was a calm, well-behaved eight-year-old with a normal attention span and level of achievement. Her customary breakfast consisted of a big smoothie and whole grain toast with real butter. She usually made her own smoothie by putting in the blender (with her mother's supervision) half an orange or apple, half a banana, a sprinkle of lecithin, a teaspoon each of wheat germ, brewer's yeast, and raw honey, one-fourth cup of skim milk or soy milk or live culture yogurt, and a tablespoon of sunflower seeds or coconut. Whirled about fifteen seconds, the smoothie came out creamy and "really good," according to the mother.

The difference in the two breakfasts? The first one was entirely processed and artificial (dead) and the second almost entirely raw (natural, alive), totally nutritious, delicious and health giving.

There are classrooms where over half the children are reported to be taking a drug called Ritalin, which has a tranquilizing effect on them. Since all drugs have side effects, shouldn't we make every effort to spare our children a life of drug dependency, of lowered health, of being put at risk for body weaknesses that may lead to serious illnesses as they grow to maturity? All this is the result of not addressing the cause of the problem and treating only the symptoms.

The parents of these small children are the first generation product of the age of processed food, junk food and soft drinks. During their growing up and maturing years, accelerated chemical dumping (estimated in thousands and thousands of tons) in the environment (air, water, food) made pollution a universal and nearly inescapable problem. Add to that pesticides and herbicides sprayed over the already leached soils, exhausted from excessive cultivation and over-farming.

Small wonder physicians, therapists and nutritionists rarely find totally healthy children today.

Chapter Seventeen

WHAT HAPPENS TO PEOPLE WHO EAT THE WAY GOD TAUGHT?

From beginning to end, every book of the Bible has something to say that applies to nutrition. The amazing thing about the end times we are experiencing is the multitude of truths on food and eating that are being discovered and brought to our attention. Sometimes God chooses a most unlikely person, in the eyes of the world, through whom He will bring such truths to light. It is a constant thrill to be learning, day by day, these newly brought-to-light facts, couched in Scripture for mankind for, lo, these many centuries. The way He wanted us to eat is among the most oft-referred-to subjects mentioned in the Scriptures.

Not until the last century has much attention been given to the way man eats or how what he eats relates to health, disease, and prevention. But as the financial interest in and fascination for medicinal drugs greatly increases, reactions and deleterious effects on the body also greatly increase. This has spurred the interest of the general public to focus more and more on foods, nutrition and healing herbs.

Names of a few nutritionists that appeared in the nineteenth century come to mind. They were people who began to realize what unnatural foods were doing to the health of mankind. Dr. Ehret, a self-educated healer, was one. He began to observe his own sickness, how medicines made it worse, and how good nutrition made it better. His writings and teaching on natural foods, mainly vegetables and fruits, gained wide recognition here and in England. Only recently have they been republished. Ellen B. White, another nutrition person, considered by some to be a prophetess, wrote in the late nineteenth and early twentieth centuries of the efficacy of natural foods on health. Her books continue to circulate, especially among the Seventh Day Adventists, whose natural, mainly vegetarian diet is credited with their having the longest lifespan of any group of people in the United States.

Fortunately, a great number of people follow the all-natural, live food way of eating. Since I myself live in like manner, I can vouch for their statements. In glowing terms, I can help to confirm the effectiveness of this way of eating *for health, high energy, ready enthusiasm, an enduring inner joy, an anticipation for each new day, a nearly tireless body, a feeling of good will toward man, a calmness, and an abiding peace.*

When a person feels good and has energy, he can handle stress and receive it as a challenge. There is nothing greater then believing God, following His will, and living in health and joyous function of body, mind and spirit for coping with life and its many stresses.

Without exception, those I know who have adhered to or made the turn-around in their "eatstyle" and lifestyle daily extol the merits of a living food or mostly living food diet. They are amazed, thrilled and grateful for the extra energy they have, the smooth-running of their physical beings, the clarity of their minds, the improvement of their memories, their uplifted spirits, the closeness they feel to their Maker. Even in their "downs," most agree, they are not submerged, overwhelmed, defeated. Their physical strength holds and their abiding faith in God sustains them. Knowing they are following His instructions about food and taking care of their bodies as well as keeping God's other commandments brings them through the "downs" to the "ups" in triumphs great and small.

All through the ages there have been philosophers and people with questioning, incisive minds who recognized the overwhelming importance of appropriate nourishment. Moses realized the influence of food on the health and function of the body and mind, God having chosen Moses to record His teachings to mankind. Isaiah, in prophesying the coming of the Messiah, wrote, "*. . . Behold, a virgin shall conceive, and bear a son, and shall call his name Immanuel. Butter and honey shall he eat, that he may know to refuse the evil, and choose the good*" (Isaiah 7:14–15). Raw, unstrained honey and fresh, raw butter are known to be brain food and soothing to the nerves. Fresh, unheated butter contains essential, *essential* oils which help to oxygenate and revitalize the body. Oils are also able to transport nutrients and micro-nutrients to body tissues and increase body energy. In fact, there is an oil called

129

Helichrysum that can be rubbed on the skin to improve the nervous system and the brain's synaptic firing of electrical impulses from one nerve to another. Oils can change electro-frequencies and balance and raise energies in body systems.

Oils, among the most ancient of medicines, were a significant part of the pharmacopoeia of the priest-physicians among the Hebrews and were much used in Egypt four thousand years ago. Today scientists have found that oils have the highest frequencies of all medicines. Measured by kilohertz (kHz), the body operates between a range of fifty and seventy-five kHz. Disease has a frequency of fifty-eight kHz on down, cancer being forty-two. To fight disease, many products are used. For doing so, drugs have a frequency of zero to ten kHz, herbs have a frequency of fifteen to twenty-two kHz, and essential oils have a frequency of seventy to 320 kHz.

According to this information, essential oils are the most effective of all these products. Having this information available, we begin to understand God's reason for giving Isaiah the prophecy about Jesus eating butter and honey. The essential oil in butter is not only for protection and treatment against disease but for stability, good mental function and steady nerves. Honey has a multiplicity of micronutrients for every phase of the body's function, including the electrical system whose center is the brain. God cautions us to eat butter and honey, these two marvelous foods, *in moderation*. Again, we see how the information in the Bible has, in many instances, quietly waited for mankind to discover, verify and utilize its vast and accurate knowledge.

According to the Scriptures, oils were respected above all curative substances and were used for both physical and spiritual purposes. Natural oils were used in religious rites to anoint (set apart as sacred), because they were soothing, healing, pain relieving and curative.

In speaking of his people, Isaiah wrote, *". . . They have forsaken the Lord, they have provoked the Holy One of Israel unto anger. . . . ye will be revolt more and more: the whole head is sick, and the whole heart faint. From the sole of the foot even unto the head there is no soundness in it; but wounds, and bruises, and putrefying sores; they have not been closed, neither bound up, neither mollified with ointment [oil]"* (Isaiah 1:4–6).

"And they cast out many devils, and anointed with oil many that were sick, and healed them" (Mark 6:13). *"Is any sick among you? Let him call for the elders of the church; and let them pray over him, anointing him with oil in the name of the Lord"* (James 5:14).

Chapter Eighteen

🌱

PARASITES—
THE SILENT EPIDEMIC

A parasite is anything living *in* you or *on* you by taking its food *from* you, whatever its size, visible or microscopic. That makes all things living in or on you parasites, be they virus, bacteria, amoebae, roundworms, flatworms, or tapeworms.

What, you may ask, have parasites to do with nutrition and the Bible? Where there are foods and people, there may be parasites. And what we eat has a great deal to do with parasites.

Not until the last few years has much attention been given to parasites. They were little *thingies* that lurked mostly in third world countries around the equator. Just maybe they were in our country in rodent-infested garbage dumps and rare areas of filth in or near a rundown city, or on an animal farm. So we thought.

As for their connection with Bible text, they are repeatedly spoken of in both the Old and New Testaments. Because of interest in prophecy today, overlooked facts are emerging and being verified daily. According to medical, Biblical and Webster's dictionaries, pestilences are plagues, epidemics of any infectious disease, which definitely includes parasites.

When we hear the term parasite, we usually think of the larger ones, from tapeworms to amoebae. But in this book parasites include the full range of the things, from the tapeworm down to the virus, the smallest of the lot. The round worm parasites—hookworm, threadworm and pinworm, and the flatworm (tapeworm and flukes)—go through several stages in their lifetime, both inside and outside numerous areas of the body. For instance, the fluke, the most disturbing of the worms, goes through five cycles to get to the sixth, the adult stage. Recent research has discovered that the adult stage of the fluke (flatworm) is in most cancers and in several other degenerative diseases, as well as in many people without these problems. If the body receives solvents from food processing and/or most shampoos and hair and skin products, the other five stages of the fluke can develop and proliferate. In fact, four kinds of fluke are found in humans.

How do we get parasites? Wherever dirt and filth exist. On unwashed fresh plants, vegetables, fruits. On doorknobs and by petting cats and dogs. (Please don't ever kiss them!) Pollutants all around us can invade the body via foods, beverages and the air we breathe and from products applied to the skin. Usually there is some toxin, slight or great, at least for some people (those who have a low immune system) which may cause a rash or dry rough skin, low energy, headaches or abnormal eye function. The list of problems caused by chemicals and other toxins that allow parasite infestation goes on and on. The presence of toxins in our bodies makes us easy prey to these microscopic, voracious invaders. In much the same way, other pollutants besides dead things, like solvents, toxic metals, molds, physical toxins such as dust, asbestos, fiberglass and smokes of all kinds, leave us vulnerable to parasites.

For instance, PCBs (polychlorinated biphenyls), banned from use in transformers, are now appearing in commercial soaps and detergents! Perhaps the most subtle, insidious pollutants are the chemicals used in products. Every household may have a product with a label warning about some toxin in it. Lawn and garden pesticides and herbicides, fertilizers, automobile fluids, paints, varnishes, waxes, bleaches, detergents, fabric softeners and so on, usually have toxic substances in them. An article that came out in a health journal recently reported nearly ten thousand chemicals in use today. Ingesting even a small bit of almost any one would mean a hasty trip to the hospital. Toxins weaken the immune system and leave the body vulnerable to all kinds of parasites, which literally move in and take over.

There is an often overlooked condition in the body that naturally protects us from ingested parasites. That condition is production of ample stomach acid (hydrochloric acid). To have sufficient acid to digest proteins—all proteins and not just animal source proteins—we need to eat natural uncooked starches, which is in all kinds of root vegetables. Sprouted grains and seeds, eaten mostly uncooked, are also good sources. When these starches are chewed *sufficiently*, they are mostly digested in the mouth. The digestive hormone ptyalin is well generated by chewing and, when swallowed, stimulates the production of stomach acid. And when the stomach acid, necessary to digest the proteins, is as high as it should be, ingested parasites are killed. That is probably why healthy raw-food vegetarians who know to eat all essential foods are little troubled by parasite infestation.

What can we do about our polluted world? God provided medicinal plants, cleansing herbs and foods to keep us healthy. If we do not alter these foods, they will give us such a good immune system, such a clean body, that parasites are resisted.

In conquering colon cancer, where parasites do exist, I followed God's instruction as closely as it was possible for me to do. Genesis 1:29 and Revelation 22:2 became my daily commitment, my guide and the basis for my hope—and assurance—that I was with God in my healing and He with me. My morning prayers started with Psalm 91:1: *"He that dwelleth in the secret place of the most High shall abide under the shadow of the Almighty."* That prayer included another awesome promise*: "Bless the Lord, O my soul . . . Who satisfieth thy mouth with good things [foods]; so that thy youth is renewed like the eagle's "*(Psalm 103:2, 5).

To understand this second Scripture fully, one needs to know the story of the eagle. This magnificent bird mates for life. In old age, he and his mate fast and molt, staying close to their nest until early spring. Then, with new feathers starting to grow, they forage for tender shoots of plants for a cleansing diet to bring about their rejuvenation. As their bodies finish the cleanse and the new feathers are fully grown back, their youth is renewed and they procreate for several years more. (This is the secret of their long active life.)

When I had a severe case of pneumonia in my sixties and nobody but my husband, God and I believed I could get well, God revealed to me this Scripture. I claimed it and repeated it every day, believing with all my heart and rejoicing for the hope it gave me. God kept His promise of renewed youth. Years later I still feel young, as I exercise vigorously each day and walk from one to three miles four days a week. I enjoy abundant energy, a clear mind, and a closeness to my Lord that is most precious. I also claimed Psalm 91:1. I do dwell "under the shadow of the most High." What an awesome place to be!

Parasites have infested the majority of us. But there are effective, natural ways to rid ourselves of them. Those ways are through powerful herbals, some of which are so powerful that they kill viruses and bacteria, even those which invade the cells. They are natural, God-provided herbals, like garlic, for example, known and used effectively for thousands of years and spoken of in the Scriptures. When the Egyptians built the pyramids, they allotted each slave laborer garlic to keep him strong and disease-free. To this day eating a clove or two of raw garlic daily is known to be an immune enhancer, a heart and circulation protector/maintainer, an anti-oxidant, and an anti-parasitic. (But garlic contains a toxic substance, to which some are allergic. Again, moderation may be a key warning for eating the powerful herb.)

For centuries cayenne has protected eaters from parasites, stomach disorders, heart attacks, paralysis and strokes and has enhanced the immune system. But only if taken raw. Cooked cayenne has lost its effectiveness. (When seasoning foods with cayenne, add after cooking and when the food is slightly cooled. Raw cayenne does not give heartburn or indigestion.)

To learn and to know about problems is to be forewarned. Headlines in the last few years have made us aware of some parasite problems and how universally prevalent they are. Some people call them "uninvited guests." My friends in Colombia where we once lived call them *habitantes* (inhabitants).

In 1993 a fast food company in Seattle served undercooked hamburgers that caused several deaths and hundreds of cases of infection from *E. coli* bacteria. That same year another parasite called *Cryptosporidium parsum* in Milwaukee's water supply caused 400,000 people to suffer such disabling symptoms as diarrhea and stomach cramps. Other cities have also had their water supplies contaminated with the cryptosporidium. Some cities gave out an alert to boil the water. Others did not, with the result of general illness and some deaths.

In the spring of 1995 the New England journal of medicine published the report of a study on cryptosporidium, which showed the parasite to be widespread and a real problem. It can infect especially those who have a weak immune system.

Very few people talk about this subtle, insidious threat to our health today. Few physicians are cognizant of the problem or can cope with it because of outdated tests, resulting in poor diagnosing. Since parasites are the basis or contributing cause of many illnesses such as muscle and joint aches, nerve and brain damage, gastrointestinal disorders, chronic fatigue and immune dysfunction, the public should be alerted about them. Parasitologists variously estimate that from 40 percent to 60 percent of us in the United States have some kind or kinds of the hundreds of varieties of parasites known to infest the earth.

Why is this so, you may ask? The reasons for the nearly universal prevalence and steady increase of the unwelcome *habitantes* are many. They are mostly related to our world as it is today near the end of the twentieth century:

- The common condition of a low immune system
- The increase in global travel, with American tourists and others visiting the farthest corners of the earth.
- Immigrants and refugees from every known para site-infested area of the world.
- Contaminated water
- Polluted air
- Household pets
- Overuse of antibiotics
- Foreign and "different" foods (e.g., undercooked animal product foods)
- Day-care centers
- Increase of AIDS
- Promiscuous sex

What can we do about this awesome specter? There are a number of things. Consult a parasite specialist. Inform yourself about parasites. There are at least two recent books on parasites with a lot of how-to instructions and sources: *Guess What Came to Dinner: Parasites and Your health,* by Ann Louise Gittleman, and *The Cure for All Diseases,* by Hulda Regehr Clark. They both give programs for eliminating parasites. People can do these programs for themselves.

You will learn about tests for parasites. If you have symptoms and wish to rid your body of them naturally, you will be informed on how to go about it. There are cleansing programs. The first step is a plan to include in the diet delicious, wholesome and natural foods, supplements of multi-trace minerals, enzymes, vitamins and natural oils in moderation, like virgin olive oil.

God's pharmacopoeia includes many plants that destroy parasites. In the food realm several stand out as being effective. For generations native Mexicans have used fresh papaya and pineapple (for the protein-digesting enzymes, papain and bromelain) to eliminate worms. My Mexican friends say a handful (about one tablespoon) of fresh raw pumpkin seeds first thing in the morning, well chewed and chased with a little water, and taken for a week or two will eliminate common worms. They skip a week then repeat the procedure just to be sure.

The list of vermifuges (worm-ridding agents) is extensive—garlic, ground almonds, radish roots, onions, carrot tops, fig extract, raw cabbage (well chewed), raw cabbage juice, blackberries, the seaweeds nori and kelp and Corsican seaweed tea. There are many herbs that help to rid and to protect from parasites: sage, male fern, black walnut hull, wormwood, clove—the list goes on and on.

A group of scientists and herbalists spent much of their lifetime putting together an herbal that they say (and time has proven to many) kills all parasites and all viruses and bacteria except pneumonia and the new, mutated tuberculoses bacillus. It is made up of eleven natural herbs and some trace minerals. As with all of God's remedies, it causes no side effects and is compatible with foods and other herbs.

The popular old proverb, "Cleanliness is next to Godliness," takes on new meaning. Today, more than ever, our very lives depend a great deal on cleanliness. The cleaner our home environment, our food, our kitchens, our hands, the more disease resistant and disease avoidant we are.

Under the fingernails is a most notorious area for harboring disease germs. We need to scrub with soap, brush and water before eating or handling foods. Parasites have difficulty living in a well-oxygenated area. They like grubby, filthy, dark, unventilated hideouts.

The "silent epidemic" of parasites is obviously one of the major plagues of today. People don't talk about parasites. They don't like to think about them or admit they exist. Few even believe these pathogenic microorganisms could ever infect or infest them. Yet parasitologists, the Center for Disease Control, and physicians and scientists on the cutting edge of today's health care world observe that outbreaks of parasites are increasing with devastating results all over the world and throughout our country. Parasites are present in, and some say causing, all cancers. They cause and exacerbate many other disorders. Everyone needs to be aware of them and their menace.

The hope of all of us is in realizing there are ways to combat parasites. First, they cannot infect a healthy body (an environment where they cannot multiply). A physician of oriental medicine, Andreas Marx, explained disease proliferation as an imbalance of the body's terrain (pH, oxidation factor, and mineral balance).

The bottom line in the condition of our bodies is our immune system. We enhance it by a lifestyle of nutrition that includes natural minerals, vitamins, enzymes, oxygen, herbs, exercise and faith. Keep in mind, God is committed to protecting us from end time plagues, diseases and epidemics *if* we keep all His commandments. Here are His promises:

"He that dwelleth in the secret place of the most
High shall abide under the shadow of the Almighty.

I will say of the Lord, He is my refuge and my fortress; my God; in him will I trust. Surely he shall deliver thee from the snare of the fowler, and from the noisome pestilence. He shall cover thee with his feathers, and under his wings shalt thou trust: his truth shall be thy shield and buckler. Thou shalt not be afraid for the terror by night; nor for the arrow that flieth by day; Nor for the pestilence that walketh in darkness; nor for the destruction that wasteth at noonday. A thousand shall fall at thy side, and ten thousand at thy right hand; but it shall not come nigh thee. Only with thine eyes shalt thou behold and see the reward of the wicked. Because thou hast made the Lord, which is my refuge, even the most High, thy habitation; There shall no evil befall thee, neither shall any plague come nigh thy dwelling. For he shall give his angels charge over thee, to keep thee in all thy ways. They shall bear thee up in their hands, lest thou dash thy foot against a stone. Thou shalt tread upon the lion and adder: the young lion and the dragon shalt thou trample under feet. Because he hath set his love upon me, therefore will I deliver him: I will set him on high, because he hath known my name. He shall call upon me, and I will answer him: I will be with him in trouble; I will deliver him, and honour him. With long life will I satisfy him, and shew him my salvation" (Psalm 91).

Chapter Nineteen

SHOULD WE FAST?

A book about nutrition as it is taught in the Bible would not be complete without a chapter on fasting. Since the Bible does not often mention fasting, either in the Old Testament or the New Testament, believers have tended to ignore it. Yet one statement alone powerfully indicates we should fast. Jesus said, *"Moreover when ye fast . . ."* (Matthew 6:16). Notice that Jesus said, "*when* ye fast," not *if* ye fast. By those few words He made it unquestionably clear we were to fast. It is an established part of our walk with Him. Jesus himself fasted, and for several profound, far-reaching reasons. If we are to truly follow God, we must fast as part of our life.

The physical reason for fasting is to cleanse the body of residual debris, waste and toxins. When too much accumulates, the performance, the function of the body and the mind is slowed down, impeded, curtailed. The spirit is dampened, leaving the emotions vulnerable to stress and upset. After a time, breakdown in health may occur, then sickness, disease and even death.

Before the time of Christ the Jewish people fasted twice a week for one meal on Tuesdays and one on Thursdays. Early Christians, used to the custom, also fasted two days a week. However, they changed the days to Wednesday and Friday, the days Jesus was arrested and crucified.

When animals the world over get sick, they fast until they are cleansed and feel well. They readily sense when their body wastes are eliminated. Then and only then will they begin to eat a little grass and drink water.

One time our beloved cat, Tigerpaw, got sick with a temperature of 108 degrees. The vet advised putting him away. We chose to bring him home and pray. He lay on the grass by the garden lily pool for eight days. The only real movement that I saw, other than his getting up to eliminate occasionally, was a weak movement of a paw as he lay flat on his side. I didn't see him even drink water.

The morning of the ninth day he chewed a very few blades of grass. Later he drank water, not from the dish I provided, but from the lily pool, a clean pool where goldfish and water plant life abounded. Through that day and the next, he ate only grass and drank water. That night I gave him a small dish of fresh raw milk that by morning was gone.

Tigerpaw quickly regained his strength and full activity on the raw foods I provided. He lived four more years to a good age without ever being sick again.

Many people, including a great number of physicians, view fasting as starvation. Biochemists have observed something quite remarkable that takes place in the fasting person. The body recycles cast-off cells. These minute amounts of nutrients are enough to keep the body functioning at a quiet, slowed-down level while it struggles at the all-encompassing task of getting rid of the toxins and the waste. For this reason, the fasting person must curtail his/her activities and rest as much as possible. Ideally, the faster should be alone most of the time, doing only mild exercise if there is sufficient strength, avoiding strenuous work and stressful situations, and enjoying a cancellation of business and social contacts. In other words, the faster should take it easy for the length of the fast and a day or two beyond.

People always ask, "How long should I fast?" A good rule-of-thumb is, "Until you feel good." If, as a few do, you feel good all through the fast, then the answer may be from three to nine days. The reason these people feel good is that they are actually quite healthy, with a minimum of body wastes and toxins to eliminate, or the person is overweight or obese, with body reserves that allow the energy to continue. In that case the body may even feel better without the "strain" of having to cope with food that it does not really need. Actually, the body is on vacation, functioning with little or no responsibility for all those extra daily chores of digesting, absorbing, eliminating and suffering myriad interruptions to its life of purposeful activity.

Unfortunately, the "happy fast" may not be for most fasters. The more physical problems, sickness and disease the person has been experiencing, the more troublesome the fast. Not infrequently I hear, "I'm not sick. I just have these pesky allergies." Well, allergies indicate problems and given time, problems become sickness and eventually degenerative disease.

Questions continue to arise. Why undergo a fast for problems? What can a fast do? How does it work? A fast can relieve and eliminate many problems by the cleansing out of body toxins. It can reveal the cause and by so doing help to diagnose the basic problem so that the therapist, the physician, or the person himself may know and treat the cause rather than the symptom.

To explain how a fast works in general everyday terms and analogies, let's take an example from nature: a stagnating pond. The life in that pond, the frogs, the fish, the tadpoles, the aquatic plants, are having a difficult time surviving. Not only is the water full of bad bacteria, slime, slush and rot, but the food supply (water insects) for the small animal life has become scarce. Any good nutrients we might add to help improve the pond for the fish, frogs and tadpoles might help sustain their lives, but those additions would not solve the problem of the stagnating water of the pond.

In order to improve the whole situation, we have first to clean out the debris that is clogging the flow of fresh water into and out of the pond. Then we have to flush out the polluted water itself until all is clean. Then and only then do we add some nourishment along with a continous flow of fresh water for the life in the pond.

At the end of a fast, the faster needs to start in the morning with diluted fruit juice, a few ounces at first, then in two hours start increasing the amount to a glassful by late afternoon. By night or early the next morning a small meal of all-natural foods is in order.

A fast is a cleaning out process, when a person ceases to add to the stagnant, overloaded body. During the fast the body's cleansing out abilities are freed. Debris—toxins, waste materials as dead cells, accumulations of undigested foods, bacteria, mucous, etc., loosen and bit by bit, flush out. The immune system gets a chance to houseclean in this vacation from daily defending, protecting and battling. The enemy of the body is mostly overcooked, processed foods, bad water and beverages and overeating, along with the consumption of sprayed and irradiated produce.

All this positive activity in the body may have a temporary negative effect on how we feel. It can make us downright sick. My best, most understandable example is myself.

Many years ago when I was sixty years old I lay at death's door, according to several doctors who watched me mysteriously deteriorate to severe gastroenteritis in spite of all their ministrations, medicines, and methods. One of them advised me to go to a fasting clinic on the Oregon Coast. The other doctors thought he had suddenly turned to quackery, and I thought he had lost his marbles. After soon realizing that no other modality had been suggested, and after praying to our faithful and caring Father, my husband and I gave in to the idea of fasting. There was no other hope in sight. Immediately we drove down the coast to the clinic.

I was fasted eight full days and nights. Upon entering the hospital, I was examined and diagnosed as having twenty-five symptoms. No other physician had ever listened to me like this fasting physician, a pediatrician/allergist. I was miserable when I entered the hospital/clinic, but I was more miserable twelve or so hours into the fast. After a milk-of-magnesia, potassium/bicarbonate "purge," I was given fresh, pure mountain water and encouraged to drink often and much. In addition, the doctor brought a shaker of pure, untreated, mined sea salt and told me to lick a little bit out of the palm of my hand now and then, to keep from dehydrating during the fast.

Never in my life before or since have I spent such an unrelieved time of misery. My legs had to be kept moving, they were so full of a creepy-crawly feeling, later named restless legs, a symptom of severe hypoglycemia. I could not sleep. I could not read. I could not listen to music. I suffered a severe headache and copious amounts of painful stomach and intestinal gas. I alternately chilled and perspired. I had a most difficult time being civil to my precious, supportive husband who read to me, brought me the news, quietly tried to chat with me, brought me flowers and a beautiful negligee. I bit my tongue to keep from biting the wonderful nurses who wore no makeup, perfume, or cosmetics of any kind because I could not tolerate the odors.

The morning of the fourth day I awoke from a brief sleep feeling well. The doctor came and said I looked quite good. "But," said he, "we'll wait until evening to see whether or not you go back into withdrawal from foods."

So that's what I was suffering from! Withdrawal. Later I learned that food withdrawal can, in severe cases, be as painful as withdrawal from alcoholism, drugs, or habitual nicotine. Mine was severe. My heart went out to all sufferers of any kind of addiction. Many, for whatever reason, never get out of it because the way is too painful, too miserable. I could thoroughly understand why.

By noon that fourth day I was back into the hell of withdrawal, this time more unbearable than ever. During the next four days I experienced a playback of nearly every sickness, every pain I had ever gone through, from the "growing pains" of early childhood, scarlet fever, frequent, upset stomach and headaches, through the pains of childbearing to the suffering of major surgery, double pneumonia, and bone-breaking accidents. The intense part of each severe pain playback lasted no more than an hour, but what a time!

Early in the morning of the eighth day I slept soundly for about four hours, the longest and best sleep of the entire fasting ordeal. The doctor came by as I opened my eyes and sat up. "You really look good," he greeted me. "I feel great," I said. Although he seemed pleased, he added words of caution. "We'll wait until evening to see if you return to withdrawal. Then we'll try the first food." His words could not dampen my spirit. "I feel so close to my Creator," I said, not knowing which "side" he was on. "We all do after a cleansing fast," he said with such enthusiasm I knew he was a believer in the Lord.

What joy that day was! I had come through the longest, the worst valley of my life. I had childlike energy, enough to shampoo and arrange my hair, to give myself a manicure and a pedicure, to read the Bible, to walk about my large room filled with early September sun. My thoughts were crystal clear, my eyesight sharp, my hearing able to detect and separate the sounds of birds, insects and the breeze in the trees of the forest just outside my hospital room. My sense of touch was so keen I could identify the several fabrics of the clothing in my suitcase and the bed linens with closed eyes. I could sniff like a bloodhound, my sense of smell was so restored. But most of all, I could concentrate, think things through, give my full attention and devotion to God through Whose Son I was made whole.

Fasting is all-important for ridding the body of toxins, disease and residual matter from undigested foods. It's the quickest way I've ever found to radiant health. The blood becomes clean and the body is restored. As important as the fast is what comes after it—the food we start eating and the lifestyle we go into.

If the faster's goal is to discover the cause of his allergies and sickness, a program of one food every four hours is worked out. At this point, a small amount of food is the way to go since the body has been at rest and will not tolerate a sudden meal of large quantities. In my case I was first given an organic banana with specific instructions to chew and chew and chew until the bite was liquid in my mouth. One small banana satisfied me. The pulse, taken in twenty-, forty-, and sixty-minute intervals afterwards showed no acceleration, which would have indicated bananas caused me a problem. But bananas were okay for me. Great! The Lord be praised!

In four hours I was given a small bowl of cooked cracked wheat. Sixty minutes later my pulse had increased twenty-four beats a minute, and in the next twenty minutes it reached 120 per minute. Another hour and my energy was gone. I lay on my hospital bed exhausted. A lab person took blood and soon came back with the report. My blood sugar level, which should have been at a fasting level of at least eighty-eight, had dropped to forty-two, down from normal in two hours' time. I was *really* allergic to cooked wheat. It was a great contributor to the fatigue that almost daily had been requiring bed rest. Later I learned that 90 percent of the population in the USA is allergic, to some degree, to cooked wheat—breads, rolls, pies, cakes, doughnuts, pastas, flour tortillas and any processed product containing wheat. I also learned from my allergist-physician that cooked, refined carbohydrates like white flour and sugar contribute the most to the bad cholesterol (LDL). The body is going to make cholesterol because every cell needs it. If we eat natural carbohydrates, the body makes the good (essential) cholesterol. If we eat bad carbohydrates (white flour and sugar), the body makes bad cholesterol.

For the next three weeks I was given a single food for each meal—fruit, vegetable, seeds, nuts, grains. Out of thirty-six foods only eleven did not give me a reaction. Most of the other twenty-five gave me a separate symptom: diarrhea, constipation, stomach cramps, arthritic pain, sore throat, spots before my eyes, headache (one in the top of the head, another an all-over headache so severe the doctor identified it as migraine), nausea, bursitis-type pain, stomach ulcer pain, swollen ankles, swollen fingers and eye bags, and little blisters in the throat, like grains of sand. In all, I experienced twenty-three allergy symptoms.

With the eleven foods I could eat and the probability of one more in our freezer at home (blueberries), I was allowed to go home. What a wonderful time it was! My slender body had given up nine pounds. (One pound weight loss a day during a fast is about the average unless the patient is very overweight and/or has water retention at the beginning of the fast).

I felt wonderful and had energy. After a few weeks on the rotation diet of one "good-for-me" food each meal every four days (twelve foods in all), I gained weight and strength. Of course I had learned what fabrics I could not tolerate, what household products I had to throw away for their toxic odor, and what gave me a problem out in the world that I needed to avoid the best I could. We had to gut the house of carpeting, wall paper, oil heating system and polyester, among other things.

God made it clear to us that without His way—the fasting way—I could not have known the cause of my many problems, nor could I have overcome all the disease my body harbored. It revealed to me His way to eat, His way to treat the body and maintain the maximum health He intends for me.

Let me say that fasting will not cure all disease. It's not the way I got over cancer of the colon or Addison's disease or a staph infection in the lungs. But by the very pronounced symptoms that specific foods caused after the fast, we learned the cause of many things I suffered, including arthritis, ulcers, tachecardia and colitis. Later, fasting nine days brought me out of pneumonia three different times. I am humbly grateful for a gracious God Who guided me through these experiences for my own recovery and to gain the knowledge to tell others.

Fasting can be recommended for many but not all people. One needs to consult a physician versed and experienced in fasting. There are books written on fasting to help reasonably healthy people who wish to fast. The average person usually gets to feeling well after a three- to five-day fast.

My healthy husband fasted five days for the knowledge and the experience. The first day he had no problem except some hunger in the evening. The second day he felt less well and was not hungry at all. The third day he felt worse. The fourth day he felt good for the most part, experiencing an occasional brief time of weakness and once a headache for an hour or so. But the morning of the fifth day he felt good, in high spirits, and with energy and clearness of mind. He kept his commitment to drive nails in the new addition to our church that first week of his vacation. Only a few times did he have to sit down to rest or let a dizzy spell pass. He was much impressed at the physical, mental, and spiritual renewing he experienced from having fasted.

Following his suggestion, we chose to fast one day a week, beginning Sunday evening and lasting to Monday evening dinner. We gave up Sunday night supper and breakfast and lunch on Monday. Many people fast one day a week, some for their health, some for their prayer life and a closer walk with Jesus. But since we are "body, mind and spirit," we learned that the fast furthers the purpose of each. In fact, we added that dimension to our life—a weekly fast—and found it wonderfully rewarding, increasing the dimensions of our life and service to our Creator.

Chapter Twenty

God's Last Promise

K nowing the truth is mind expanding. It gives a feeling of security, of completeness. It contributes to peace in our life and radiant joy deep within. A classic example of one of these truths is knowing that body, mind and soul-spirit are all a part of our wholeness. They cannot be separated lest the person become dysfunctional in first one way, then another.

How interesting it is to note the order in which the components of our being are listed when referred to or identified in the Bible. Always first is the physical—the *body.* Then comes the *mind,* which is the liaison between the body and the *soul-spirit.* Last is the *spirit.* First God formed the body (physical being). Then He breathed life into it, which activated the *body* and the *brain* with their separate yet interlocking functions. Lastly He anointed the being with *spirit,* the master gift for His supreme creation.

All through the Bible, when the natural and the spiritual are mentioned, they are in that order, the natural and the spiritual, the body, mind and spirit. *"It is sown a natural body; it is raised a spiritual body. There is a natural body, and there is a spiritual body"* (I Corinthians 15:44).

As believers, how can we allow ourselves to neglect one or the other? Any slighted part of the wholeness of man—body, mind and spirit—cripples, distorts, nullifies the complete function. It lessens, over a period of time, the effectiveness, the accomplishments God has in His will for us. It leaves unfulfilled the purpose He designed for each of us.

Nurturing the body with natural *plant food* to maintain the mind with constructive *thought food* and to provide the spirit with *faith food* (the Word of God) leads to effectiveness, regeneration, growth, achievement and the fulfilled purpose God planned in the beginning.

Too often He is blamed for our setbacks, be they accidents, victimizing occurrences, "mysterious" and "unaccountable" illnesses, financial vicissitudes, emotional problems, mental and spiritual aberrations, or whatever. Yet many times—and I do sincerely believe, during my long life of trial and error, the *majority* of times—we can rightfully take the blame for the greater share of the problems we suffer.

Let's take for an example what contributes to some of the problems we suffer—the lack of sufficient exercise in our world today.

The people of Bible times walked everywhere. To celebrate the Feast of the Passover in Jerusalem, the majority of them walked from the surrounding villages, towns and countryside to the Holy City. Some walked days to get there. Not only walking but also working daily at all sorts of tasks provided essential exercise. The men cultivated the fields.

They lifted, carried, handled animals, cut down trees, cleared stones out of fields, built rock walls, and did many, many more tasks that called for great strength and endurance. The women lifted and carried heavy clay pots of water for their households, carried their babies everywhere, cleaned their houses with brooms they made themselves, bathed their children, helped harvest crops, and performed countless other tasks. They were strong, active and mostly disease free. It does not compare at all with today where technical and mechanical labor-saving devices have replaced many health-enhancing activities. Actually, we were designed to walk and do physical work.

This brings us back to the law of cause and effect, referred to earlier. Of course there are exceptions. God, because of our prayers and those of others, does intercede. He sets things right or He walks us lovingly through the "dark valley," teaching, revealing, instructing, sustaining us in the knowledge that leads to wisdom.

That's how I reached the light after many years of struggle, searching and believing through the darkness of severe and multiple illnesses. I had not cared for the temple of my soul—God's temple. All else in my earthly existence came first—ambition, education, career, marriage, family, intellectual achievements, self-fulfillment, enjoyment, travel, friendships, and so on. Finally, at death's door through neglect of nutrition, exercise, rest, spiritual focus and maturing, I realized man's way (prescription drugs, clinics, hospitals) was truly destroying me. In total surrender I turned to God Who amazingly heard my desperate outcry. Incredibly, when I was at death's door He put joy in my heart and hope in my spirit. Then in an awesome but slow turn-around, He guided me through the neglected, strange-to-me, simple yet long way back to health. He also showed me His promise that, joy of joys, restored my youth at sixty-eight years of age. *"Who redeemeth thy life from destruction; who crowneth thee with loving kindness and tender mercies; Who satisfieth thy mouth with good things; so that thy youth is renewed like the eagle's"* (Psalm 103: 4–5).

Claiming that promise with all my heart, I followed God's eating instruction to the letter—raw fruits with their seeds and "leaves of the tree for the healing of the nations." In other words, also leaves of edible weeds, vegetables, and other trees. Modern, scientifically oriented man took a long time to discover and recognize chlorophyll as one of the most healing of substances, the ingredient in plants that gives them their gorgeous green color. Incidentally, blood hemoglobin is like chlorophyll except for one thing. Hemoglobin has an iron molecule where chlorophyll has a magnesium molecule. Interestingly, both are basic to health and healing. Both pure blood and organic, living, green plants are stressed in God's word: The "life is in the blood," and "leaves for the healing."

To be restored to health after nearly a lifetime of following the worldly way, I had to be *born again* in every sense of the word, surrendering my life to God. Changing to the Lord's way was not always easy, yet it was basically simple. God did not make things complicated in His commandments. They became complicated by my procrastination, my stumbling, my doubting, my reluctant following of His step-by-step instructions. I had to stop complaining, even a little bit. *God cannot answer our prayers when we complain.*

Little by little, in His loving, gracious patience, the way became clear. With only slightly accelerating progress, I continued, slowly gaining, advancing, learning, conquering. With each triumph, no matter how small, my joy knew no bounds. Even in setbacks—and they frequently occurred despite my efforts—I rejoiced because joy reigned in my heart. I knew Jesus, the great Healer. He is the vine (the trunk and the roots). Jesus was in me and I in Him. Of course He was "in me" and "I was in Him"! Hadn't He made that quite clear? The vine can't produce any fruit without the branch, and the branch cannot live without the sap (strength, energy, power) provided by the vine.

With each accomplishment came a bit of energy. In time, I could walk a few blocks without exhaustion and climb a stair without help. Most of all, even before I conquered severe hypoglycemia or arthritis or recovered from terminal Addison's disease (atrophy of the adrenal glands) or that killer, cancer of the colon, or the devastating chronic fatigue syndrome, I began to be pain-free and to feel good most of the time. I had to learn that even one helping of wrong food was a setback, a day or so in bed, the flare-up of hypoglycemia, constipation or diarrhea or the pain of arthritis or the haunting, deep "hurt" in the tumor area of the colon.

In several forceful lessons I learned that a terminally ill person cannot afford to take *one bite* of food that is not health giving, disease conquering.

Remember, please!

Cooked foods are not health giving.

They are simply life sustaining!

God gave us the proper instructions in what to eat—all natural, raw, living foods. The more unnatural (processed, synthetic, artificial, additive-drenched) the foods, the worse for us they are. The more we eat them, the sooner we lose our health. By carrying on with wrong eating and continuing to pollute the body, we cannot enjoy a good immune system nor can we withstand the plagues, the pestilences, the infections, the infestations, the diseases of the end times. We will surely perish from illness, which is not in God's plan for us.

However, God assures us that if we *keep His command-ments* He will protect us from the end time afflictions.

"If thou wilt not observe to do all the words of this law that are written in this book, that thou mayest fear this glorious and fearful name, THE LORD THY GOD; Then the Lord will make thy plagues wonderful [fearful], and the plagues of thy seed, even great plagues, and of long continuance. Moreover he will bring upon thee all the diseases of Egypt, which thou wast afraid of; and they shall cleave unto thee. Also every sickness, and every plague, which is not written in the book of this law, them will the Lord bring upon thee, until thou be destroyed" (Deuteronomy 28:58–61).

Cheer up! There is great promise and assurance in the next two Scriptures: *"...If thou wilt diligently hearken to the voice of the Lord thy God, and wilt do that which is right in his sight, and wilt give ear to his commandments, and keep all his statutes, I will put none of these diseases upon thee, which I have brought upon the Egyptians: for I am the Lord that healeth thee"* (Exodus 15:26).

"Wherefore it shall come to pass, if ye hearken to these judgments, and keep, and do them, that the Lord thy God shall keep unto thee the covenant and the mercy which he sware unto thy fathers . . . . And the Lord will take away from thee all sickness, and will put none of the evil diseases of Egypt, which thou knowest, upon thee..." (Deuteronomy 7:12, 15).

Then in the New Testament, under the new covenant, we find this assurance: *"Since we have these promises, dear friends, let us purify ourselves from everything that contaminates body and spirit, perfecting holiness out of reverence for God"* (II Corinthians 7:1). (Notice the order of the *physical* and *spiritual*. The physical holds first place, to bring it to special attention.)

The commandments most of us fail to keep are those that tell us to take care of our body with exercise, right eating and not overstuffing our precious stomach.

Not only is the end reward for our faith and obedience great, but the blessings of obedience to our Heavenly Father and, in turn, to us along the way, far exceed the earthly understanding of us, His children, who love and follow Him. The benefits will surprise us all!

The awesome wonder of life is our resplendent Lord God Himself, Who truly *loves* us. To follow Him in every way, all the way, is to become His vision for us—radiant in health, inspired in mind and anointed in spirit.

"Bless the Lord, O my soul: and all that is within me, bless his holy name. Bless the Lord, O my soul, and forget not all His benefits" (Psalm 103:1–2).

BIBLIOGRAPHY

Klassen, Frank. *Chronology of the Bible.* Nashville, TN: Regal Publishers, 1975.

McLean, G. S.; Oakland, Roger; McLean, Larry. *The Evidence for Creation: Examining the Origin of Planet Earth.* Santa Ana, CA: Understand the Times.

Saddler, William S., M.D. *The Physiology of Faith and Fear.* Chicago: A. C. Mclurg & Co., 1918.

Tennyson, E. T. *The Diet of Oxygen.* Jefferson City, MO: Harvest Publishers, 1956.

The Student Bible: New International Version. Grand Rapids, MI: Zondervan, 1986.

To order additional copies of
Does the Bible Teach Nutrition?
send $11.99 + $3.95 shipping and handling to:

WinePress Publishing
PO Box 1406
Mukilteo, WA 98275

•

To order by phone
have your credit card ready and call

(800) 917-BOOK